PERFECT HEALTH

THE COMPLETE GUIDE FOR BODY & MIND

BODY, DIET & NUTRITION

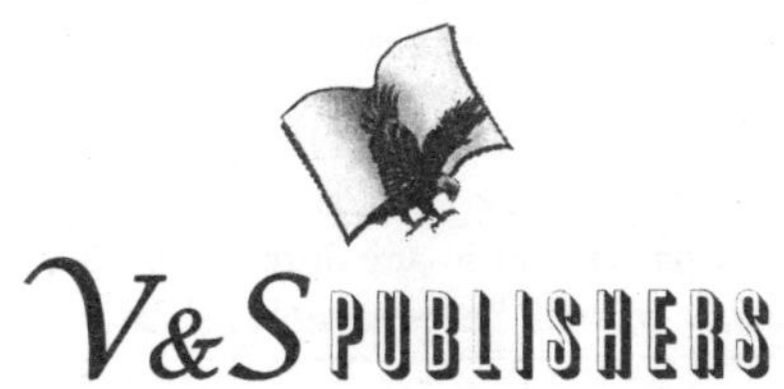
V&S PUBLISHERS

Published by:

F-2/16, Ansari Road, Daryaganj, New Delhi-110002
011-23240026, 011-23240027 • *Fax:* 011-23240028
Email: info@vspublishers.com • *Website:* www.vspublishers.com

Branch : Hyderabad
5-1-707/1, Brij Bhawan (Beside Central Bank of India Lane)
Bank Street, Koti, Hyderabad - 500 095.
040-24737290.
E-mail: vspublishershyd@gmail.com

Follow us on:  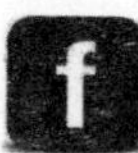 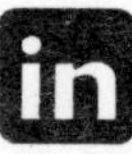

For any assistance sms **VSPUB** to **56161**

All books available at **www.vspublishers.com**

ISBN 978-93-815883-6-9
Edition 2014

Printed at : Param Offseters, Okhla, New Delhi-110020

PUBLISHER'S NOTE

According to Francis Bacon, "A healthy body is the greatest chamber of soul; a sick one, its prison." But to maintain a healthy body one must not only follow the rules of moderate health living coupled with a state of moral relaxation exercising one's judgment in meeting the strains and stresses in life but must also understand the disease process, since a proper understanding of not only the health but also of the sickness is essential in maintaining a healthy being.

The present day stress of life produces harmful effects not only on different organs of the body but also on the psyche. There is no denying the fact that both the mind and body are so interlinked that their mutual interaction constitutes equal share in the maintenance of the normal human cycle.

To live a normal healthy life one has to live life and enjoy it. Life can't be a mathematical equation of do's and don't but, put in a judicious manner; the various intricacies of a healthy and diseased body must be well appreciated. If one can understand that the road to healthy living through a life of moderation in one's habit and attitudes towards life, the task becomes much easier.

To make the task easier we present to you *Perfect Health,* a set of four books.

Book I: Perfect Health: Body, Diet & Nutrition
Book II: Perfect Health: Fitness & Slimming
Book III: Perfect Health: Health Hazards & Cure
Book IV: Perfect Health: Stress & Alternative Therapies

This set of four books is not meant to create awareness about the physical well-being alone. There are many books doing that, already. Instead, all the four books are all about creating awareness that fitness of the mind and emotions is as important as the fitness of body. And unless one works at being fit in every way, one is not likely to find true health.

To many, this would seem an unattainable goal but it is not so. The effort required to work towards an integrated health and fitness regime is hardly any more difficult than trying to balance your social and spiritual life. Where there is a will, there is a way. And so with fitness.

Perfect Health provides a complete step-by-step program of mind body medicine tailored to individual needs. The result is a total plan, tailor-made for each individual, to reestablish the body's essential balance with nature; to strengthen the mind-body connection; and to use the power of quantum healing to transcend the ordinary limitations of disease and aging – in short, for achieving perfect health.

CONTENTS

SECTION 1

Know your Body

Chapter **1**

BODY, MIND & SOUL

A body is needed for inner health and growth of the 'self'; *shariramādyam khalu dharmasādhanam*. We must have control over our senses for real health. He who has little control over his senses can hardly remain healthy. In the Gita Lord Krishna said that the sense organs wish to enjoy every pleasure. Such pleasant things are the real cause of pain. Whatever we see is mortal. A wise man will not prefer those worldly pleasures:

> ***Bhoktāram yagyatapasām sarvalokamaheshwaram***
> ***Suhridam sarvabhutānām gyātwā mām***
> ***shāntimprichchhati.***

The Gita 5:29

We aim at remaining healthy and happy; and to excel simultaneously in many fields. We usually claim to be experts, which we, ordinarily are not. The ego in us makes us the expert, and the superiority complex compels us to give advice even to real experts. We are really expert in searching out the weaknesses, and to en-cash it.

But we don't know the fundamental facts about our body, our mind, the functioning of our organs, the system as a whole; and the most important thing "The Elements". We attach little importance to them and are never shy of wasting or polluting them. When we pollute or waste the elements, we are destroying ourselves. Our forefathers were great and wise that they saved them.

Our ill health is the result of our inhuman thought and unhealthy food. We care little for our body or mind. We go for junk food and have developed unhealthy habits while the fact is that 'the purity of self depends on the purity of food, *āhārashudhhou satwasuddhi*. Purity is the only way otherwise no one will be satisfied after living a sensuous life.

Negligence and Misery

The human body is created with the elements which have a lot of influence over our body, mind and physical well being. A slight negligence can cause immense damage and generate untold misery. One can see physically handicapped people everywhere: men, women and children. Why has the number of physically handicapped grown to such dangerous proportion. It's only because of the negligence towards the life-giving and preserving elements. It will be too late; if we are not awakened now. A normal child or a normal man could be a rare sight. It will be difficult to live and behave in normal way. There is another effect of the negligence of the elements. Most of the people are behaving in abnormal fashions: mothers are killing their children; fathers are killing their sons; sons are killing their fathers; brothers are notorious in shooting their brothers; servants are killing masters and vice versa; doctors are killing, patients and guardians are killing the doctors; students are killing their teachers and teachers are beating students to death; misbehaviors are common things; wives are killing husbands and vice versa. Stop and think what is wrong with man?

Unfortunately, we are living in an age completely dominated by science and technology. Everyone is running after materialism. In this race they are losing vital elements and all important vitality. In exchange they are getting unheard diseases. We have lost contact with fresh and pure elements; sacred and divine scriptures; inner purity and spirituality. Nature and natural habits have lost their significance. Clearly, it's perversion but we are claiming it to be modernity; and that we are living a fast life; of course without life.

All the factories and machines are robbing off life, affecting health by polluting air and water; snatching away our creativity and inflicting injuries to our organs. We have lost our mental peace and equilibrium. The indecent ads are adding a lot to demolish the established norms but we are not as yet ready to awaken and be conscious; and to make our conscience the real guide.

We are breaking the structure and system on which Nature and life stand while opting for radiations which are coming to us with 'electronic equipments'. It's all because we don't heed to the teachings of our forefathers who laid a lot of stress on *Bahyabhyantar shuchih*: inner and outer cleanliness and purity. Only right type of clean atmosphere can ensure health and help in sustaining life. All of us are suffering from certain disease and most of us are suffering from chronic diseases. It's all because of imbalance in Nature and natural elements.

Controlling Body for Greater Energy

The whole universe is a configuration of triple energy or triple form or tri qualities. Human beings also have this 'tri' in possession so human life is tri-basic or tri-farious or tri-facial: a combination of three distinct qualities, form or energy called: Body; Mind and Soul. But these three are distinct, not replaceable by one another.

There is another tri; tri-guna, tri-qualities: *Tamas, Rājas* and *Sattva* that deals with lower, middle and higher character; mundane, royal and pure; physical, mental and spiritual. It shapes the mind, character, growth and progress of a person. It determines one's yearning and also the changes that occur.

But the tragedy is that most people fail to use their physical power; don't realize the power of the mind; and barring a few don't even think about the soul and its abundant power and divine significance.

The Body

We always grow from inside. Everything grows from inside. All the outer growth is from inside. All separate entities have come out of one entity. The space is the greatest creation. There won't be dimensions without space. Only the outer growth is seen and the inner growth is missed. The hands, legs or nails and skin come out because of the subtle and concrete growth from inside. They are not outer parts but are called so. They are as much inner parts as heart, lungs, kidneys or brain. They grow and function in accordance with the system or systems. They are not stitched from outside. They become longer, thicker or more solid only from inside. We always grow from inside.

The growth seems to be in fraction or parts but it is not so. We are divided in infinite fractions. Modern scientists call them cells, which is given the power and agility to grow on its own, as Brahman divided His self into infinite fraction for both subtle and concrete growth. So, every existing thing or being is like Brahman, has the subtle and concrete forms and spirit, soul or self; and works and grows; and has purpose and pursuits to follow. We are all like Him; we are all like Brahman. The Rishis knew it and taught us: *yat brahmānde tat pinde*; whatever is there in the universe, it is also there in the body. We don't realize and we don't think.

The existence or the God or the Godliness in existence decides the purpose or pursuit; the ways, the means and makes the self to grow, and leads the soul to enlightenment or destruction or peril.

Our Possessions

Our body is not all that we possess. Body is only the outer garb for inner life; *Prāna Tatva,* the living spirit and soul. Besides the physical body we possess an immensely powerful 'Spiritual Self'; that is life and 'I' of each person. In Indian Scriptures physical body is an instrument for realizing, spiritual body called *Ātmā* and through it the *Param Ātmā*. Usually that spiritual self resides in its pristine self. We have to find it, see it, feel it, awaken it and make it manifest. One who knows his Ātmā is in possession of a Spiritual Self; the rest do have it but since they don't know or meet or face it so they don't have the spiritual self. They are the ignorant one or they are always referred to as 'ignorant.' Ignorant does not mean not knowing the world or worldly things. Ignorance means not knowing Ātmā or the Spiritual Self.

In the words of Vivekanand: "Always think of the body as your house. The people and the world are all absolutely unreal like a dream. Always think that the body is only an inert instrument. And the Ātman within is your real nature.

Learn to feel yourself in other bodies, to know that we are all one. Throw all other nonsense to the winds. Spit out your actions, good or bad, and never think of them again. What is done is done. Throw off superstition. Have no weaknesses even in the face of death. Do not repent, do not brood over past deeds. Be āzad, be free."

Each one has a body but no one is the body. The body is not the person though it belongs to the person. The person is neither his/ her hands nor legs; neither head nor toe; neither intestine nor heart. He/ she pervades all: the whole body. As the pervading entity in the body he/ she is a soul. Each one has a soul but he/ she is not the soul. A person is both the body and the soul in it. So each one possesses and belongs to both his/ her physical self and spiritual self: *Body* and *Soul*.

Our dilemma, the dilemma of modern man is that we worry about and cater only to our physical needs and forget and ignore the spiritual need. As a result the body, wealth and luxury grow and the soul weakens and becomes empty.

Body is not life there is life in the body. We are not the body in which we are. Body is needed to foster the life force i.e. *Prāna Tatva* or Spirit, the *ātmā* or the soul to be more exact; for its growth, development, refinement and possible salvation, *Moksha*, freedom from the endless cycle of birth-death and birth or rebirth. In that sense all our birth are rebirth. Whenever we are miraculously saved, it is said to be a rebirth. For that very purpose of growth, refinement and salvation, one must keep the body healthy and fit to perform greater and wholesome deeds to take care of all sorts of life on the earth: both human and non-human. That is the purpose of life.

Chapter 2

SCIENTIFIC STUDY OF BODY

Human body has a defined structure to stand, sit, bend or lie down. The whole structure is made up of **skeletal** and **muscular** systems. The skeletal system is made up of 206 bones and muscles of different kinds are attached to it with tendons to allow the bones to move; to give movement to human body. Different types of movements allow fulfillment of all our needs.

Skeletal system acts as a shield to protect delicate organs. Bones protect the marrow and the rib cage does the same to heart and lungs; the skull protects the brain; the vertebral column protects the spinal cord; the hip bone protects the urinary bladder and womb in women.

Muscles are made up of fibres which contract and relax. Muscles equal half of the body weight. They are 640 in number and hardly work alone; at least they work in pair. Muscles push and pull. When one of the pair pulls the other relaxes.

The Digestive system performs its task in four stages: Ingestion when the food is taken into mouth, chewed, gets mixed with saliva and swallowed. The proper function of Digestion begins in the stomach as the second step when the food reaches there through a food pipe called Oesophagus; and when the enzymes are mixed and food is broken into small molecules. In the intestine the food is further broken into smaller pieces and Absorption is completed. All the nutrients are absorbed by the walls of the intestine, and then, passed into the blood stream. The 4th act is Ingestion when the undigested food particles that reach the large intestine are further absorbed and the waste is stored in the rectum from where it's excreted through anus.

The Respiratory system completes the act of taking in air, using the oxygen and getting rid of carbon dioxide, a harmful gas produced inside. Lungs are the most important organs of respiration. Lungs are situated inside the chest and are connected to mouth and nose. Here the blood gets a fresh supply of oxygen. Breathing involves two acts: inspiration i.e. breathing in and expiration i.e. breathing out.

Though Urinary and Reproductive system are important but far more important is the Circulatory system. The opinion may vary because through the reproductive system children are born and through the urinary tract the waste liquid is excreted. Each moment that we spend on the earth is made possible because of the circulation of blood throughout the body. The Heart, its main organ works round the clock and throughout the life. Death occurs when it stops functioning. The failure of any inner system can cause death. The heart beats 72 times a minute and pumps out about 340 litres of blood every hour. It's both a tough and important work. We often say, give rest to your mind. The mind may take rest, the heart won't.

Heart is made up of cardiac muscles and a sophisticated pump which pumps the blood to each part of the body. It's in the shape of a fist and divided in two parts: right and left which is further divided by a thick wall of muscles into lower and upper chambers. It is joined by the veins and arteries. The veins carry impure blood to the heart and the arteries carry oxygen-rich blood from the heart. The reverse force is stopped by valves. The blood contains red cells, white cells and platelets; and plasma.

The immune system consists of Tonsils and Adenoids which help to destroy foreign substances that are breathed in or swallowed; Thymus is in the front of chest which helps white cells to kill germs; White blood cells directly attack the germs in any part of the body; Spleen which makes and stores white cells. The Skin secretes antibacterial substances and Tears and Mucus contain an enzyme called lysozyme that breaks down the wall of bacteria.

Glands and Hormones

Our body is the greatest and most complex chemical factory. It prepares everything that it needs not in the same way as the plants do but in its own way. In the plants, photosynthesis occurs, but in human body chemicals are secreted by different glands. These chemicals are known as Hormones and the small but main factory is known as Endocrine glands. There are smaller factories also in the form of other glands.

Apart from the nutrient and water our body needs chemicals too to carry out the processes smoothly. These chemicals are made up of amino-acids, a constituent of hormones. The creator has created a grand hormone system in the body. The whole system is known as endocrine system whose foundations are the hormones and glands.

Glands are a collection of cells or tissues that remove specific substances from the blood; alter or concentrate them; and then, either release them for further use by the body or eliminate them. The functional cells of a gland typically rest on a membrane, and are surrounded by a meshwork of blood vessels. Endocrine or ductless glands (pituitary, thyroid or adrenal) discharge hormones into the bloodstream directly. Exocrine glands (digestive; mammary; salivary and sweat) discharge their products through ducts. Pituitary gland secretes more than nine hormones; and also controls most of the activities of other endocrine glands. It is controlled by hypothalamus which is located just above the pituitary gland in the brain.

The pancreas is also a part of this hormone secreting system though, it secretes digestive enzymes also. Some non-endocrine glands such as: brain, heart, lungs, kidneys, liver, thymus, skin and placenta also produce and release hormones. Thyroid gland releases a hormone called Calcitonin to maintain the level of calcium in our body. It also releases some other hormones like thyroxine and triodothyronine which affect blood pressure and increases the rate of metabolism.

The pineal gland secretes melatonin hormone which affects reproductive development, and daily physiologic cycles. Alpha cells in pancreatic islets secrete the hormone insulin in response to a low concentration of glucose in the blood. On the other hand Beta cells in the pancreatic islets secrete insulin in response to a high concentration of glucose in the blood. Improper function of pancreas causes diabetes. Adrenals secrete corticosteroids hormone that maintain the levels of water and salts in our body. It is also maintained by kidney which releases rennin for this particular purpose. Ovaries release oestrogen and progesterone hormones which bring changes in girls and prepare them for motherhood while testes release testosterone which brings changes in boys and help them to mature into manhood.

When hormone production reaches a certain normal or necessary level any further secretion is controlled by important body mechanisms to maintain the level of hormone in the blood. The whole body acts on the theory of balance. Too little or too much of the secretion of hormones is harmful to the body. Wrong secretion will cause trouble, for example, if male hormones start secreting in a girl; then hairs will start growing on her body; her sound would change and become deep; the skin will become somewhat rough; Imbalance in secretion may result in faster or slower growth. A child can grow very tall. In any case, some sort of abnormality develops.

Major Hormone Producing Sites

Glands	Location	Hormones produced	Effect
Hypothalamus	Above the pituitary	Releasing and inhibiting purpose	Coordinates the working of hormones and nervous system.
Pituitary	Middle of the brain	Growth Hormone	Regulates body activities and growth.
		Thyroid Stimulating Hormone TSH	Controls the Thyroid.
		Anti-diuretic Hormone ADH	Controls level of water.

Glands	Location	Hormones produced	Effect
		Follicle stimulating FSH & Luteinising LH	Stimulates production of sex hormones in males and females.
Thyroid	Below voice box	Thyroxine (T4) Tri-idoththyronine (T3) Calcitonin	T3 and T4 affect the speed of chemical processes; Calcitonin regulates the level of calcium.
Adrenal	Above the kidneys	Andrenalin Noradrenaline Cortisol	Take care of level of water, salts & minerals; Help to cope with stress and disease.
Pancreas	Near the liver	Insulin; Glucagon	Controls level of glucose.
Kidneys	Abdomen	Rennin	Controls water & salt.
		Erythroprotein	Speed up manufacture of Red-cells in blood.
Stomach		Enzyme	Speeds up digestion.
Ovaries	Lower abdomen	Oestrogen Progesterone	Stimulates puberty.
Testes	Lower abdomen	Testosterone	Stimulates adulthood.

Growth Hormone GH; also called Somatotropin; is peptide hormone secreted by the anterior lobe of the Pituitary gland. It promotes growth of bone and other body tissues by stimulating protein synthesis and fat breakdown for energy. Excessive production causes gigantism; acromegaly; or other malformations; while lower production results in dwarfism; dramatically relieved if GH is given before puberty. Genetic engineering techniques now permit large-scale production of adequate amounts of GH for that purpose.

Chapter **3**

PARTS OF BODY

Skin, the outer protection, has two layers known as: epidermis and dermis. The delicate nerves and tissues lie beneath them. Epidermis has hard and tough cells which get flattened, die and are transformed into a material called Keratin, which is finally shed as tiny scales. In the dermis are sweat glands and ducts. The skin is water-proof and heat proof. It will not dry up in heat or melt in the rain. It protects from harmful radiations; acts as a shield against injury; conserves heat during winters and cools body during summer. It keeps the internal temperature constant.

Muscles make our movements possible through contraction and expansion. There are three types of muscles: Striped muscles are composed of tissues, and are called voluntary for they are under the control of the brain. Each major muscle consists of several bundles, made up of a number of fibres. Smooth muscles consist of long cells tapered at both ends. They are found at the lining of gut and the walls of the arteries. They are called involuntary muscles for they are not in the control of the brain. On the other hand they are responsible for the muscular construction. They work on their own. Cardiac muscles are similar in structure to voluntary muscles but the fibres are thick and short; and form a dense mass.

A cell is a unit in which all life activities take place. The basic structure of every living being is composed of cells. Each cell lives its own life and at the same time makes it possible for the living being as a whole to carry on its life-activities. The useful matter in the cell is the protoplasm, which carries on all the processes necessary for life. It takes in food and oxygen, changes food into living matters, gives out waste, repairs its worn-out parts, and forms and produces itself.

There are plants and animals ranging from one cell to millions of cells. The most complicated cell structure is of human. There are animals of lower order and lesser cells also. Cells are organized in group of cells of a particular kind to perform a particular type of work. They are called tissues as bone tissues or muscle tissues etc. When several tissues are combined to perform a given task then it's called an organ.

In human body there are five important types of cells: Epithelial cells make up the skin, the glands and line the body vessels. Muscle cells make up all the three kinds of muscles. Nerve cells make brain, spinal cord and nerves. Blood cells are found in the blood and lymph. Connective tissue cells make up the framework tissues of the body. Cells are the building blocks.

In the circulatory system the great wonders are the **Arteries** and the Veins. They are blood vessels. Blood is sent from the heart through arteries that carry pure blood to various parts of the body; and through veins impure blood comes back to the heart. The right auricle receives blood from the body. The heart or the auricle contracts and blood flows into the right ventricle. The ventricle contacts, it pumps blood into the lungs. The left auricle receives blood from the lungs and passes it to the ventricle. Within seconds the process is over; but it continues incessantly to keep us alive. In that process and in the split seconds the blood is purified and sent to the whole body as well as the impure blood is collected from the whole body. The whole circulatory system works on its own.

The cells live and work separately and in conjunction with others. So do the tissues. In this way all the organs work independently and also as a part of the complete system. The functions and activities of each organ are co-related and synchronized. A slight deviation will cause illness.

Brain is the most important organ of the body. It controls and regulates the functioning of whole body. All other organs are equally important. What can the brain do, if blood is not supplied to it? A momentary lapse of blood supply will paralyse the brain. Man will be alive but the brain will not be functioning.

Brain is located in the skull, well protected because it's very tender and subtle. It has three main parts: Forebrain,

Midbrain and Hindbrain. The anterior part is the forebrain which includes the olfactory lobes (the centre of smells); and cerebral hemisphere (the seat of intelligence). The midbrain includes optic lobes, the centre of vision. The hindbrain is the posterior part which includes cerebellum (co-ordination centre) and the medulla oblongata (centre of involuntary actions) Medulla Oblongata lies behind the spinal cord. All the functions are controlled by the brain. The brain is connected to each part of the body with nerves which form a delicate nervous system. It receives the messages and passes the orders which are immediately sent to the organs for necessary action.

The brain and the spinal cord form the central processing unit of nervous system. The brain stem, which links the brain with the spinal cord, is a part of the hindbrain. Sleep and wakefulness are located in the brain stem.

Liver, weighing between 1.36 to 1.81 kg, is the largest organ in the human body. The proteins, both of vegetarian and animal origin, form 'raw proteins'. Liver makes them acceptable to the body first by breaking them down. It manufactures certain proteins on its own such as Fibrogen, the blood clotting protein. It turns carbohydrates into two forms: one is "instant energy" in the form of glucose and the other is "stored energy" in the form of glycogen. It produces a hormone which can store excess sugar present in the blood as glycogen. Fats are also turned into different forms by liver as subcutaneous layer and act as insulation and shock absorbers. It produces bile (pitta) which is a thick yellow or greenish fluid and it neutralizes the acidity of partly digested food in the intestine so that enzymes can continue to work there. It is also a storage organ. Several vitamins, iron (removed from blood pigment) are stored in liver. It also neutralizes poisons and wastes.

The urinary system is a part of the cleaning system and consists of two kidneys, ureters, urinary bladder and urethra. Kidneys are situated at the back of the abdominal cavity, one on each side of the vertebral column. They are made up of a large number of 'caoated tube-shaped filters' called nephrons. They extract nitrogenous waste material and excess water from blood and form urine which passes to the urinary bladder via ureters. From there it's expelled through the urethra by contraction of muscles. The removal of such waste material is essential in all living organisms. Normal function of kidney ensures good health.

The other important cleaning organ is the **spleen** which is an integral part of the lymphatic system. It lies just below the diaphragm, at the top of the left side of the abdomen. It's one of the main filters of blood. It removes the old and worn out blood cells and also abnormal cells. It plays a major part in getting rid of the harmful bacteria. It also makes antibodies. Enlarged spleen is an indication of some disease in the body.

A gland is an organ which produces a chemical substance that regulates the metabolic activities of the body. There are two kinds of glands: Exocrine glands which have ducts leading to the outside; and Endocrine glands which are ductless. Sweet glands secrete sweet through coiled ducts to the surface of the skin. Digestive glands secrete digestive juices in the stomach and intestine. Salivary glands produce saliva. They are all exocrine glands. Endocrine glands secrete hormones which are chemical messengers released directly into the bloodstream and are used to control metabolic activities such as growth and development. One of the most important endocrine glands is pituitary gland which is situated in the brain. It is called the master gland. Thyroid gland is a special large bi-lobed gland situated behind the larynx (voice-box) in the neck. It secretes throxin hormone that contains iodine. It controls general metabolism of the body and accelerates the production of energy and consumption of oxygen. Excessive secretion increases body temperature, fat is depleted and the body loses weight. Reduced secretion will cause hair-loss and swelling of tongue and vocal cords.

Blood in itself is a wonder. It absorbs, carries and distributes all the elements and energy to each part of the body.

Blood is a tissue that has different kinds of cells in pale liquid called plasma. Red cells are red due to the presence of pigments called haemoglobin and carry oxygen. White cells are fighter cells. It fights against germs and other foreign bodies. It helps in maintaining a constant temperature in the body. Blood contains antibodies. These are proteins manufactured by the body that fight against foreign substances called antigens. When an antigen enters the body, it stimulates the immune system to produce antibodies (The immune system is the body's natural defence system). The antibodies attach, or bind, themselves to the antigen and inactivite it.

Eyes, the organs of vision are very delicate organs. Eye-balls are protected in a socket with eye-lids, eye-lash and eye-brows. The outer layer of the eye-ball has three layers: the outermost layer is tough and elastic. It's opaque at the back and is called sclera; and it's transparent at the front and is called cornea. The middle layer supplies blood to the eye. The innermost layer is the retina which is an extremely delicate tissue. At the centre of the eye is a circular opening called the pupil which is a hole in the middle of iris. Iris is just behind the cornea. The pupil appears black because no light is reflected from it. The lens is immediately behind the pupil. The space between cornea and eye lens is filled up with a vision liquid called 'aqueous humour'. The light coming from an object enters the eye through cornea. When we see an object, the light-waves entering our eyes are focused on retina by the lens.

The lids of our eyes are our built in wind-screen wipers. The lids are made up of folds of skin, and they can be raised and lowered by certain muscles. Our blinking provides automatic lubrication to the eyes. The eyelid applies suction to the opening of the tear gland and takes out some of the fluid. This prevents the eyes from drying out. The tears contain an antiseptic which kills germs. It protects against bacteria. The eye-lids are directly in contact with spinal cord. So, when suddenly an object approaches our eyes, the eye-lids are closed in a reflex action.

Chapter **4**

JOINTS

There would be no movement in animals including human beings without the joints. On the other hand, in trees and rocks there are such joints which won't allow movement.

In animals, the bones are attached to voluntary and involuntary muscles. Hence, joints move in them either at the dictates of the brain or on their own volition. Evolution won't make certain organs and their parts to work on their own and others to obey 'brain' for brain is there in each living being according to their life style and needs. A great deal of scientific experiments and thought over 'the fundamental, normal, abnormal and intricate needs of the shape, nature, food habit and the availability of the needed things' are needed for making such joints (for that matter, the whole body and each organ) which must be studied in detail (most of the important organs of human body will be discussed here and now) to prove the point beyond all reasonable and unreasonable doubts.

In human body the joints allow the bones to glide smoothly with very little or no friction. The cartilages cover the bones so that they don't rub against one other. Moreover, a whitish fluid is secreted by the joints, called the Synovial Fluid which acts like an oil in a machine to reduce friction.

There are 'four main types' of joints.

1. **Ball and Socket Joints** are found in the shoulders and so it has the greatest range of motion for man. Other joints in the body don't have that much of movement
2. **An Ellipsoid Joint** is another kind of joint. It is an egg shaped surface that fits into an elliptical cavity. Wrist joint is the example. It allows only elliptical movement and stops circular movement.
3. **Hinge Joint** the third type of joint in which the bones can be moved to and fro in one plane.

4. **Rotary Joint,** the fourth type is the joint at the base of our skull. It moves in such a way that we can turn our heads. Other rotary joints are found at the elbow.

Besides these four main joints there are many other joints like the Saddle Joints in which the bones can move in two directions. The example of this kind is our backbone which can be bent and straightened.

It's very easy to say that the life evolved out of 'nothing' it's very difficult to accept or deny 'rationale' behind such indispensable joints which can make 'Men'; and only they can make man. How is it that each cell or each seed will grow in 'this' or 'that' particular pattern. The evolution in itself will not think of the days ahead and works to be accomplished after the complete growth and maturity or during the old age. It will not think of which animal will need jelly like body and which will need a shield like cover.

Joints are very important. Joints can be taken care of by correct posture, rhythmic and steady movement by avoiding undue pressure on the joints.

Chapter **5**

GENETICS

DNA, deoxyribonucleic acid, is a nucleic acid that is the chief constituent of the *chromosomes* carrying genetic information, in the form of *genes*, necessary for the organization and functioning of living cells. The molecular structure of DNA was first proposed by JD Watson and FH Crick in 1953.

The DNA consists of a double helix of two strands coiled around each other. Each strand is made up of alternating pentose sugar (deoxyribose) and phosphate groups, with an organic base attached to each pentose group. There are four bases: adenine (A); guanine (G); cytocine (C); and thymine (T). The bases on each strand are joined by hydrogen bonds which are always bound in the same way; A always binds with T; and G with C. During replication, the strands of the helix separate and each provides a template for the synthesis of a new complementary strand; thus producing two identical copies of the original helix. This special property for accurate self-replication enables DNA to duplicate the genes of an organism during the cell divisions of growth and production of cells for the next generation.

If it's evolution and self-replication of cells then how is it that each man has a different DNA?

Chromosome

Chromosomes are thread like structures that carry the genetic information of living organisms, and are found in the nuclei of their cells. Chromosomes consist of a central axis of DNA with associated RNA and Proteins. Before cell division, the long filamentous threads contract and thicken, and each chromosome can be seen as two identical threads (which are known as chromatids.) joined at the centromere. The chromatids later separate to become the daughter chromosomes.

Chromosome number is characteristic of a species. For example, a human cell has 46 chromosomes comprising 22 matched pairs (which are called autosomes.) and two sex chromosomes. A human sperm or egg cell has half this number of chromosomes. Abnormal numbers or parts of chromosomes often lead to abnormalities in the individual concerned. Down syndrome, called mongolism, is caused by the presence of an extra copy of genetic material on 21st chromosome, either in full or in part.

Genes

Genes is a unit of the hereditary material of an organism that provides the genetic information necessary to fulfill a single function. The term gene was first coined by WL Johansen in 1909.

Genes were initially conceived as a string of beads comprising of the chromosome; they were later defined as lengths of chromosome that were physically indivisible during the exchange of chromosomal material that occurs during meiosis. Alternatively, a gene was defined as the shortest lenth of the chromosome that could undergo mutation.

However, with the discovery of the structure of DNA and the molecular basis of heredity, a gene was re-defined as "being a functional unit (cictron) corresponding to a specific sequence of the genetic code." Structural genes code for individual polypeptides while regular genes control the activities of structural genes. Genes are means by which information for the organization and function of living cells is carried by DNA and RNA molecules. Evidence for the nature of genetic code was provided in the 1960s by the work of Crick, Nirenbeg, Khorana and many others.

They found that the basic symbol of the code was a sequence of three consecutive bases mentioned earlier as DNA or RNA. The different triplet codons or sequences couls specify the 20 or so amino acids commonly used by cells synthesis; and give start and stop signal for the process.

Investigations in many species have shown that the code seems to apply universally.

RNA

RNA, ribonucleic acid, is a nucleic acid that is important in the synthesis of proteins in living organisms. In some viruses RNA is the genetic material. Structurally, it's similsr to DNA but usually occurs as a single stranded molecule with the sugar ribose and thymine of DNA. There are three main types of RNA, most of which occur in the cell cytoplasm: ribosomal (r) RNA; messenger (m) RNA; and transfer (t) RNA.

The genetic code in DNA contains information necessary for protein synthesis. This code is transcribed into a strand of mRNA and carried to the risomes which are small cytoplasmic particles. There it is translated into a particular polypeptide chain. The amino acids making up the protein are brought to correct positions in chain of tRNA.

Peptide is a chemical compound comprising of a chain of two or more amino acids linked by peptide bonds (-NH-CO-) formed between the carboxyl and amino groups of adjacent amino acids.

Polypeptides, containing between three and several hundreds amino acids, are the constituents of proteins. Some peptides are important as hormones e.g. ACTH and as antibiotics e.g. bactracin, grad mecidin.

Mitosis

Mitosis plays its own part. It's the process by which the nucleus of a somatic cell (i.e. any cell that is not a germ cell) duplicates itself exactly, producing two daughter nuclei with chromosomes that are identical to those of the parent nucleus. This nuclear division involves the separation of the two chromatids of each chromosome, which move apart to form two groups at opposite ends of the cell. In the final phase each group becomes enclosed in a new nuclear membrane. After this the cytoplasm usually divides to form two new cells. Mitosis occurs in most animals and plants during the normal growth and repair of tissues.

In this way meiosis, which is the process by that the nucleus of a germ cell divides prior to the formation of gamets, such as sperm, pollen or eggs; plays its own part to influence the whole life. Through meiosis the formation of four eggs or sperm cells from one parent cells take place in two divisions, each of which is divided into several phases.

Chapter 6

SUNSHINE AND OUR BODY

The Sun gives life to all living body. If you wish to remain healthy take the shelter of the Sun. There are numerous diseases which are cured by the Sun.

All the seven rays (colours) of the Sun give seven different types of energy. The therapy done through the Sunrays is called Colour Therapy; Chromotherapy or Chromopathy.

Sunshine destroys certain fungi and bacteria that settle on the skin. It causes the whole blood cells or phagocytes to become more active. These are the cells which attack germs in our body and help us keep healthy.

When the Sunlight strikes the skin, certain substances are sent into the blood, which gives the muscles new tone. The muscles become tense, and, thus, we can work better. In fact, our nervous system gets a kind of 'charge' from Sunlight. We feel stimulated and want to move about. Another major importance of the Sunlight is that it produces vitamin D in our body. The ultraviolet light helps in the production of vitamin D. Balanced exposure to Sunlight is good but excess exposure to it is harmful.

Pouring water from above the head in front allows the sunrays to enter the body and strengthen many inner organs; and also keeps the skin healthy and shining. So, after taking bath, when the body is almost uncovered, most of the Indians worship Sun by pouring water in that particular fashion. Although, it's a part of rituals; it is scientific and a very healthy and beneficial habit.

It's always advised to take sun bath (almost naked) during morning and evening hours when the sunrays are not very hot.

Elements in Body

The human body is made up of the five elements: Soil; Water; Fire, Sky and Air.

The bones and the marrow in bones; muscles, cartilages and the skin are made up of the earth elements; meaning that the earth is made up of different substances. Those substances have been used to create the body. Man belongs to the mammal group and all the mammals are warm blooded animals. Human body has a lot of heat which helps him digest the food, change it into energy, and make adjustments with the outer heat. The average temperature of a human body is around 95 degree Celsius. Two third of the body is made up of water. Air is easily inhaled and exhaled through nose, mouth and wind pipe. It gives the much needed oxygen to purify and revitalize the blood and also helps in excreting out the waste in the form of air or gases. Human body has a lot of space for the expansion and contraction of different organs. It helps not only in the growth of the organs but also in the 'intake of food and water' and excretion of waste materials from the body through kidneys and anus.

The human body is made up of different elements. It contains over twenty different chemical elements. Oxygen is the most plentiful element in the body. Oxygen together with hydrogen forms water. Water makes up nearly two third of the body weight. The body of an average person needs about five litres of water every day. We drink water or fulfill this need in different ways but equal amount of water is discharged from the body every day.

The body has a good amount of carbon in it. Much of this carbon together with oxygen and hydrogen makes up fat and sugar. Carbon, hydrogen, oxygen and nitrogen form the body's vital proteins. Large amounts of calcium and phosphorus are also present in the body. It contains about one and a quarter kilograms of calcium. The body also contains sulphur, iron and about 30 gms of other metals.

The whole of our body is divided in voluntary and involuntary actions and functions. Out of the 640 muscles that we have some are under our control and some not. Those under control are called voluntary; those that don't are called involuntary.

The muscles work in pair; when one expands, the other contracts. It's not only with the muscles but it's true to each part and organ of our body. They perform voluntary and involuntary actions and functions; they obey or disobey us according to the circumstances, need and the type of order.

SECTION 2

DIET AND NUTRITION

Chapter **7**

FOOD FOR HEALTH

Ways Means to be Healthy

Right living is essential for achieving a long and healthy life. Irresponsible living is the breeding ground of diseases, pain and suffering. It burns out the highly sensitive organs. Yoga is always fruitful in keeping the body healthy and pollution free. The inner body has been created in such a way that it equips it for survival under unfriendly and difficult circumstances. If we treat our body carelessly and roughly we would weaken it on one hand and the mind will degenerate on the other.

Food

Food and diet is important. It's our basic need. It must be balanced both in quality and quantity. One must eat everything, but not daily, and never too much. A bit of many things will be sufficient. The things that grow in a particular season only should be taken to make one's diet balanced. *That is what the people say, advise; and that is what people don't follow.* Food must be taken only when the first intake has already been chewed. In general condition food is digested in about four hours. One should not keep ones stomach empty. Something must be eaten after every six hours. Only such things should be eaten which can be digested. Undigested food weakens the body.

Food Chain

What is food chain in general terms is the food web in its real form. It seems to be a very simple system but in fact it's very complicated. It's not easy to know which living organism depends on whom for food; because each living being depends on more than one thing, object, organism for its food; and because the leftover of one being is the food for another; and his leftover for yet another; and so on. That is what makes it complicated.

Food chain or web can be treated as eternal food exchange among a series of living organisms. They are all associated in a feeding relationship; or even dependent on each other for food and thus for survival. The most wonderful thing is that one organism feeds on the other just below it in the chain of numerous food-material and innumerous organisms.

Most commonly the green plants are in the middle to balance each other. They feed on dead organisms and decomposed things; and almost all living beings: man, animals, birds, insects, and pests; depend directly or indirectly on them. Plants and plant products are eaten by herbivores; which are in turn consumed by carnivores.

Many parasitic organisms and plant parasites are also part of the chain; and different food chains are interconnected to form a food web. Other food chains are based on decomposers: organisms that feed on dead organic remains of plants and animals.

We are destroying the food chain in an indiscreet manner. We are throwing the garbage in drains which deprives the animals from their much needed food. When in the drain the cereals and other things decompose they give bad smell and give birth to germs for the growth of diseases. In that process we stop the flow of the drain. There are some simple questions; civic sense may follow the question. Are we human beings? Are we intelligent? Have we wisdom? Should we survive?

In the food web some 'beings' eat their off-spring; snakes for example; and some off-springs feed on their mothers; crabs for example. Are we not like crabs and snakes?

Food Preservation

The treatment of food to prevent its deterioration and to maintain its quality and nutritional value is called food preservation; and the process through which it's preserved is called food processing.

Breakdown of food tissues is caused by enzymes, either contained within the food or produced by micro-organisms such as bacteria, yeasts and fungus which grow in the food. These organisms also produce unpleasant and sometimes harmful substances. Oxidation and dehydration contribute to spoil food. So, food preservation is needed.

The principle of food preservation is to alter the condition of food so that the activities of micro-organisms are stopped. One of the oldest methods is drying or dehydration used for meat, vegetables, cereals, milk-products etc. Freezing is now widely used for both industrial and domestic food preservation. Heating kills micro-organisms and is the principle of pasteurization, sterilization etc. Further growth of micro-organisms is prevented if food is sealed in airtight containers, such as cans (canning) or bottles (bottling). A wide range of chemicals is added to food to inhibit microbial activity but this process is very dangerous, as all the norms are hardly maintained and the chemicals turn poisonous. Smoking has also been used to preserve meat and fish. Sodium benzoate, propionates, nitrates, nitrites, sulphur dioxide and sulphites are used by modern food industries that enhance colour and texture to food. This makes the pulp of the fruits and vegetables tasteless and unhealthy; even poisonous.

Food-poisoning

Food poisoning is an acute illness arising out of eating contaminated food. Vomiting and diarrhea are the usual symptoms. Salmonella is the bacterium that most commonly causes food poisoning which is known as salmonellosis. The symptoms begin between 12 to 24 hours after eating the contaminated food. Another kind of food poisoning is due to a toxin (poison) produced by staphylococci. The symptoms occur within one to three hours after taking the contaminated food. Clostridium bacteria may also cause food poisoning. The most severe form is known as botulism. It's a rare and serious form of food poisoning from the food containing toxin produced by the bacterium clostridium botulinum. The toxin affects the cardiac and respiratory centres of the brain, and results in death by lung or heart failure.

Physical Labour

Physical labour is the most essential requirement for good health and strength. Muscles and bones will not grow strong; breathing will not be regulated; blood will not be purified; strain will not be tolerated and hands and legs will not get powerful without physical labour. One must indulge for four hours (may be two hours in the morning and two hours in the evening) in such works in which sweat start flowing. There is no question of ego or wealth, it's the need. After looking at own or others' de-shaped body one must opt for physical labour. Gyms will not do for usually gyms are indoor activities while outdoor activities are needed.

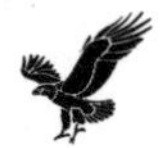

Chapter **8**

THE FOOD

Grains

The seeds of cultivated cereal grasses; grains are a mainstay of human nutrition. They are naturally high in complex carbohydrates and fibre and low in sodium and sugar. Most are also low in fat and a good source of niacin, thiamine, riboflavin, vitamin B6, and some minerals. Although grains do provide protein, it is incomplete protein, lacking certain essential amino acids.

The seeds of cereal grasses-consist of three parts:

- The bran, or layered outer coating
- The germ, the embryo of the new plant
- The endosperm, which feeds the germ.

Each section contains different nutrients. The bran contains B vitamins, minerals, protein, and most of grain's dietary fibre.

The germ has fats, B vitamins, minerals and protein.

The endosperm, the largest section of the grain, is mostly starch, with some protein.

A whole-grain product contains all the components of the grain. A refined grain product consists mainly of the starchy endosperm. In removing the bran and germ, the refining process trips away most of the valuable vitamins, minerals, protein, and fibre in grains.

White flour and other refined grain products are often enriched, a process that restores a few of the lost nutrients but not the fibre. Some grain products are labelled as 'fortified', meaning that they have had nutrients added to them, which were not there to begin with. A fortified breakfast cereal, for instance, contains added vitamins and minerals.

Vegetables

Vegetables are useful sources of minerals, vitamins and fibre, and also provide some polyunsaturated fat. Vegetables in the diet may actually protect a person against cancer. A number of surveys have shown that people who eat plenty of fresh vegetables, such as lettuce or celery, are less likely to get stomach cancer. The importance of vegetables in the diet for prevention of cancer has now been demonstrated in animals, and has led to the discovery of a new class of substances, which protect against cancer.

A study showed that several members of the *Brassica* family, including cabbage, Brussels sprouts, turnips, broccoli and cauliflower, caused the protective enzyme to be made in the liver. Spinach, dill and celery are equally effective, but the vegetables varied in their effect according to their freshness, variety and the soil in which they were grown. The study was also able to identify the actual chemicals in the vegetables, which cause the protective enzymes to be formed. This was an organic chemical called indoles. It was found that citrus fruits (oranges and lemons) contain chemicals called flavones, which, like indoles, cause the protective enzymes to be formed in the liver.

Other plant product may protect against cancer. Beans and seeds are rich in plant proteins called lentils, which increase movements of the bowel, they have been found to protect animals against cancer in laboratory experiments. Beans are not only important in being a low-fat substitute for meat; they also seem to have a positive effect in lowering cholesterol, and it does not seem to matter what type of beans is eaten. Cucumber has a very cooling effect on the body. It is rich in potassium, due to which it helps combat fatigue and muscle weakness. Cucumber juice is also very effective in treating hyperacidity. It prevents the accumulation of uric acid and is therefore beneficial to those suffering from gout and rheumatism. Cucumber juice is a skin cleanser and is more effective when taken along with carrot juice.

Several different experiments have shown that onions or garlic contain chemical substances which alter the ability of the blood to clot. This has led to the suggestion that onions and garlic are valuable in preventing the formation of blood clots, which are a cause of coronary heart attacks and strokes.

To get maximum benefit from the vitamins in vegetables, cook briefly so that they are still a little crisp to the taste. Overcooking destroys the vitamin C in vegetables and washes other nutrients into cooking water, which may be discarded. The water used to cook vegetables may also be utilized as stock for stews so making sure that minerals and vitamins are not lost.

Fruits

For years, we have known the efficacy of fruits and in India. Fresh fruit juices and vegetable juices have potent cleansing properties. They help the liver in its job of cleansing the body of toxins. Fruits can be easily digested and offer a pleasant break from eating calorie laden, difficult to digest meals. Over consumption of animal foods such as chicken, mutton, meats, and high fat cheese, make the blood acidic. Fruits, with their alkaline nature, help to balance the over use of such foods. Ayurvedics strongly recommend intake of fruits to neutralise the acidic nature of other foods.

Fruits also have a natural laxative effect: When eaten in the raw form they are rich in enzymes - for example, papaya contains papain which helps to digest proteins; pineapple contains bromalain, which is excellent for digestion, and prevents gas or flatulence.

Fruits are also rich in anti-oxidants and bioflavinoids: which help boost immunity and delay the aging process. Some fruits are specially known for their healing properties.

Apple: It contains pectin, which helps reduce cholesterol. Apple juice is a potent liver cleanser and is also used to remove gallstones. It has a cooling effect on the body and reduces heat related ailments like heat boils and is therefore the ideal during the summer. Since pectin also has stool-binding properties it is useful in controlling diarrhoea. It can sometimes cause constipation in some people.

Banana: It is rich in potassium and thus useful in reducing blood pressure. Because bananas have a lubricating effect on the intestines, they are useful in treating ulcers. Slightly raw banana is used to treat constipation. It is also very easy to digest and so it is an excellent food for the aged as well as small children.

Watermelon: This popular summer fruit has many beneficial properties. It is not only cooling, but is also a natural diuretic. Watermelon is very alkaline in nature; it has a soothing effect on the stomach and prevents biliousness. It is the best thirst quencher and is beneficial for those suffering from kidney problems and urinary tract infections. Watermelon helps dehydrate the body and is low in calories and high in nutrients.

Pineapple: An enzyme called bromalain, which is present in this exotic fruit is very helpful in digestion. It soothes the effects of excess bile, cools the stomach and is effective in relieving abdominal pain and gas. It is especially good for people suffering from heart disease because it contains vitamin C and manganese that help in preventing the formation of blood clots. Pineapple is also a natural diuretic which helps prevent water retention in women.

Oranges: Oranges are synonymous with vitamin C due to which this fruit gets a lot of good publicity. It is also fairly rich in calcium. It has a highly acceptable flavour and is a hot favourite among dieters. It helps prevent colds and increases immunity. It can be digested very easily and should be given to children as well. Oranges if eaten with the pith, help prevent constipation. Orange juice is a good source of calcium and vitamin C for children. It helps prevent gas and aids digestion.

Mango: is also a good source of beta-carotene, which is converted to vitamin A in the body. A medium sized mango can provide the vitamin A supply for a week and unlike vitamin C, this can be safely stored in the body.

Each fruit contains its own set of known and unknown anti-oxidants, which work together to protect cells against number of diseases. Therefore, to maintain a good health, we should ingest a wide spectrum of fruits and vegetables every day as part of our regular diet.

Chapter **9**

FOOD PYRAMID

Everyone talks about eating the right food but what is generally ignored is the right amount of food that needs to be eaten.

It is important to know which type of food is right for you and stick to a nourishing diet that takes care of all the nutrients that are required by the body. The best way to find out what is required to be eaten every day is to have a look at the 'Food Pyramid'. The pyramid provides a basic food pattern that should be taken in each category. The basic principle being, that a variety of food should be eaten each day, to get the right nutrients and right number of calories in order to maintain the optimum weight. Following the 'Food Pyramid' guidelines will ensure that you never go wrong, as far as nutrients are concerned.

There are five major food groups and no single food group is more important than the other, nor can it be replaced with another. For healthy eating, one requires food items from each group.

Level one – Right at the base of the pyramid, are food items that come from grains. They provide carbohydrates along with other essential nutrients. Foods like bread, cereals, rice, pasta, etc., should form a bulk of our diet. Care should be taken to ensure that they are in their unrefined form, for maximum benefit. Hence, it is better to have brown bread instead of the white one, bran included flour instead of the refined one. Needless to say, eating the good old chapatti is any day better than eating bread, especially the white bread.

Level two – Just above it, the pyramid section is divided into two parts. This level includes foods that come from plants - vegetables and fruits. Importance of these two elements can never be undermined as they form a vital requirement of all diet. (More information on vegetables and fruits is given elsewhere in this chapter).

As we all know, a major part of vitamins and fibres come from this group. For an ideal balance, one should take about 3-5 servings of vegetables and 2-4 servings of the fruits.

Level three – The third level is again divided into two parts and the foods that are included in these parts come mostly from animals. Milk, yoghurt, cheese and meat, poultry, fish, dry beans, eggs, and nuts form this level. These foods are required for a healthy nutrition because they provide the essential elements like protein, calcium, iron and zinc. Just two or three servings of these are enough for a healthy diet.

Level four – The tip of the pyramid comprises fats, oils and sweets. All kinds of dressings, fats, butter, creams, soft drinks, desserts, etc. are included in this category. These foods provide calories and hardly any nutrition so they should be used sparingly. By using these foods sparingly, you can have a diet that supplies needed vitamins and minerals without excess calories.

Related Facts

- Foods like milk and meat groups that come from animals are high in fat, unlike the food that comes from the plant group.
- Fruits, vegetables and grain products are low in fat but when they are fried, they become unhealthy. A baked potato has hardly any fat and just 120 calories, but 14 French Fries have 11 gms of fat and 225 calories.
- While keeping a tab on the sugar consumption, don't forget the sugar that is added to food, like the cereal and coffee, etc. A soft drink contains many more times of sugar than is required for the daily intake. Chocolate milk, canned fruits, cakes and pastries also add to the excess.
- Choose lower fat foods from the food groups whenever possible.

Calory Requirements

- ❑ Most sedentary women and older people require just 1600 calories every day. Pregnant women require more calories.
- ❑ For children, teenaged girls and active women, 2200 calories is quite enough.
- ❑ Very active men and women as well as teenaged boys require 2800 calories.

Food as per calories – For active women who need about 2200 calories a day, 9 servings of breads, rice, cereals or pasta would be just right. Just about 170-180 gms of meat should be enough.

Total fat should be restricted to about 73 gms per day.

For women who are moderately active and require something like 2000 calories, just 8 servings of the grain group would be enough.

Chapter **10**

NUTRITION

Nutrition is essential for living. A lot of ignorance is connected with nutrition and diet. One can eat to live or live to eat, those who eat to live are much healthier than the ones who live to eat. The idea is to eat a nourishing and well balanced diet in order to remain at the optimum fitness level. This chapter is all about the right diet and the ill effects of the wrong one.

It is essential for a person to control the diet in a manner that the essential nutrients are obtained by the body to keep it in optimum functioning level. At the same time, care has to be taken to avoid abusing the systems by loading them with harmful food elements. We need to eat a variety of food so that the body obtains all the vitamins, minerals and nutrients required by it.

Nutrients can broadly be divided into two categories - macronutrients and micronutrients

Macronutrients

Macronutrients are the foods that should form the bulk of our diet. All of the foods you eat are composed of three macronutrients:

- Carbohydrates
- Protein and
- Fat.

Some foods are primarily carbohydrate (bread); others are mainly protein, and some are pure fat. Other foods are combinations of two or all three. A slice of pizza is a perfect example. The crust and tomato sauce provide the carbohydrate, and the cheese provides protein and fat. In order to properly function, your body needs all three of these macronutrients in approximately the following ratio:

55 percent carbohydrate, 15 percent protein and no more than 30 percent total fat.

Nutrient	Calories per gram
Carbohydrate	4 calories
Protein	4 calories
Fat	9 calories

Micronutrients

Micronutrients are composed of vitamins and minerals. They are the key to all the complex reactions that take place in your body. Although they don't provide energy directly, vitamin and minerals work together to help carbohydrate; protein and fat produce energy, to assist with protein synthesis and to help keep the body functioning normally. Compared with the macronutrients (protein, carbohydrate, fat), vitamins and minerals are needed in small amounts.

Elements Needed for Well Balanced Diet are:

Carbohydrates - include sugars, starches and related substances, which are chemical compounds of carbon, hydrogen and oxygen. Plants make carbohydrates from carbon dioxide and water, using the energy from the sun. Potatoes, pasta (spaghetti etc) bread, rice, and other grains are rich in carbohydrate. Cellulose and other indigestible carbohydrates are an important part of the diet, as a source of fibre, which aids the passage of material through the bowel.

Proteins - are the essential 'building blocks' of the living cells and comprise about 12 per cent of the weight of the human body (water 70 per cent, fat 15 per cent). Proteins are made up from some 22 different amino acids. Proteins can be made by the body into an enormous variety of shapes to do various different jobs. Enzymes, the biological catalysts of the body, are all proteins and there are many thousands of them in the body-each one different. Proteins in the food are broken down by digestion into amino acids, which are then rearranged into new proteins needed by the body. All necessary protein is obtained from bread, grains and beans, although meat fish and eggs are good sources.

Vitamins - are substances needed by the body, which the body cannot make for itself from raw materials. Vitamins are only needed in small amounts, mostly as catalysts helping along vital chemical reactions. Shortage of vitamins cause deficiency such as scurvy (shortage of vitamin C), rickets (shortage of vitamin D), beri beri (shortage of Vitamin B) and others. A balanced diet contains all the necessary vitamins.

Chapter **11**

VITAL VITAMINS

Vitamin C

Probably the most well known antioxidant, vitamin C helps minimize free radical damage to the neurological system. In the presence of hesperidin, a bioflavonoid, vitamin C is an even more powerful antioxidant. It also protects other antioxidants in the body, such as vitamin E. In addition to neutralizing free radicals, vitamin C detoxifies the body, reduces high blood pressure, lowers cholesterol, and fights cancer.

Vitamin A and Beta-carotene

Both vitamin A and beta-carotene are powerful free-radical scavengers that help the skin, mucous membranes, circulatory system, and cholesterol levels. In particular, beta-carotene is very effective in neutralizing the singlet oxygen-free radical. More than 600 different types of carotene have been identified from fruits and vegetables, only a few of which have been studied. Preliminary research indicates that alpha-carotene is up to 100 times more powerful as an antioxidant than beta-carotene. Others include lutein, gamma-carotene, zeaxanthin, and lycopene, a known cancer fighter that occurs in high concentrations in tomato products.

Vitamin E

This antioxidant prevents the oxidation of lipids (fats) in cell membranes, which strengthens the outer cell layers against free radical attack. Vitamin E works best in the presence of selenium, another antioxidant, and helps protect vitamin A. Vitamin E stimulates the immune system, improves the circulatory system and oxygen absorption, fights cancer, and has a role in preventing cataracts.

Lycopene – There is no question today that antioxidants are a significant part of the important nutrients we need today to support our health. One of the more newly discovered antioxidants is lycopene. This much-hailed phytonutrient is found in tomatoes. It is actually the substance that gives tomatoes their red colour and, like beta-carotene, is a member of the carotenoid family.

Research on dietary lycopene suggests that it may lower the risk of heart attack. A five-year study of 48,000 men found that those eating ten servings per week of cooked tomato products had the lowest risk of prostate cancer. Believe it or not, their risk was only one-third that of men eating less than two servings per week. Other studies suggest that lycopene may play a major role in reducing the risk of other cancers, including cancers of the breast, rectum and colon.

And there's more. While fresh tomatoes are loaded with lycopene, cooking them makes it even easier for your body to use their lycopene. Apparently, as the tomatoes break down when they are cooked, the lycopene is more easily absorbed. Including a little fat will help, too, especially mono saturated fat like olive oil.

It is not known exactly how much lycopene one should consume each day, but based on recent studies, you would probably want to eat ten servings of tomatoes per week.

When you exercise heavily, you need additional antioxidants according to a leading researcher. Exercise stimulates your body's production of "free radicals" that attack cells, leading to long-term damage and a higher risk of cancer. To counteract the exercise hazard, experts suggest taking antioxidant supplements daily, notably vitamin E (400 IU) and vitamin C (1000 mg).

Chocolate facts – One scientist recently discovered that chocolate contains phenolics, an antioxidant that is believed to reduce your overall chances of contracting heart disease. Pure chocolate may be the best chocolate around. That's because the fat in pure chocolate usually comes from cocoa butter and cocoa butter has a high content of stearic acid, the saturated fat that doesn't hurt your blood cholesterol level. What's better for you, white or dark chocolate? As a general rule, dark chocolate is made from a higher content of cocoa butter. It also contains many phenolics. White chocolate usually doesn't have very many phenolics, but is loaded with cocoa butter. A dark chocolate bar is considered the most beneficial, followed by fudge syrup, baking chocolate, chocolate fondue, and semisweet chips.

Coffee cure - Brewed coffee seems to create hundreds of new chemicals that appear to have antioxidant qualities. Each chemical is present in only tiny amounts, but taken together in a cup of coffee, they could add up to have about the same antioxidant effect as three oranges.

Selenium support - Selenium has been found to be beneficial in the fight against free radicals, which contribute to premature ageing, among other things. Selenium is found in the highest concentrations in sea-foods, grains, muscle meats, and Brazil nuts. A multi-vitamin that contains between 70-100 mcg is recommended, but an additional supplement is not necessary. It has been recently shown that selenium can help prevent cancer.

Zingy Zinc

Just like it protects your car from rust, zinc has antioxidant properties that protect the body. Zinc is required to maintain effective levels of vitamins E and A. It is also a key ingredient in the very important antioxidant enzyme called superoxide dismutase (SOD).

Grape Seed Extract (Pycnogenol)

Pycnogenol is an effective antioxidant. Common sources are the bark of the French maritime pine tree (Pycnogenol), grape seed, lemon tree bark, peanuts, and cranberries. Research indicates that this compound may be 20-50 times more potent than vitamins C and E. besides; it keeps joints and skin supple, promoting a youthful appearance. It also strengthens capillaries, improves circulation, reduces joint pain, and protects nerve tissue.

Other Plant Sources

Several popular supplements- bilberry, ginkgo biloba, and garlic- are very strong antioxidants. Bilberry helps eliminate free radicals from capillary walls and red blood cells; it is also known to check arthritis. Its ability to improve vision was first observed during World War II when it was discovered that British pilots, who ate bilberry jam, had excellent twilight vision. Ginkgo biloba is famous for improving memory, partly because it contains antioxidants that scavenge free radicals and boost the effectiveness of vitamin C. It also improves circulation, heart conditions, and neurological disorders such as Alzheimer's disease.

Garlic contains high amounts of antioxidants vitamin A, vitamin C, carotene, and selenium and boosts the levels of antioxidant enzymes in the bloodstream. Green tea also contains a variety of antioxidants, including catechin, and is known to lower cholesterol levels and reduce blood clotting.

Vitamin Values

Fat soluble vitamins – they are mainly found in oils and fat containing foods. Since the body stores these in its fatty tissues, one does not need to eat them every day. Overdoses can be toxic.

Vitamin	Benefits	Sources
Vitamin A (retinal) Vitamin D (calciferol) Vitamin E (tocoferol) Vitamin K	Needed for maintenance of skin, mucous membranes, bones, teeth and hair; eyesight, and reproduction; may protect against cancer. Helps absorb calcium; needed for bone growth and maintenance.	Liver (especially fish liver), egg yolk, fortified margarine, oily fish, oranges, apricots, carrots, tomatoes, melons, dark green leafy vegetables. Fortified milk, dairy products, fish liver oils, fatty fish, eggs, and fortified margarine, also synthesized by ultraviolet light.

Vitamin	Benefits	Sources
	Cell growth, antioxidants Essential in production of some proteins that help in the clotting of blood.	Vegetable oils, nuts, dark green leafy vegetables, whole grain food, wheat germ. Most vegetables – especially the dark green leafy ones, eggs, cereals, liver.

Water-soluble vitamins are found in a variety of plant and animal foods. Because the body stores them in small amounts and quickly excretes excesses, they need to be part of your diet nearly every day.

Vitamin	Benefits	Sources
Vitamin B1 (Thiamine)	Helps break down carbohydrates; nervous system.	Most foods – including wheat germ and pulses, whole grains, brewer's yeast, nuts, fortified breakfast cereals.
Vitamin B2 (Riboflavin)	Repairs body tissues and helps release energy from foods.	Brewer's yeast, liver, milk, kidney, dairy products, wheat bran, wheat germ, eggs.
Vitamin B3 (Niacin)	Essential for tissue chemical reactions, needed for nervous and digestive functions.	Wheatgerm, whole grain cereals, peanuts, legumes, meat and fish.
Vitamin B5 (Pantothenic Acid)	Helps metabolise nutrients	Liver, kidney, wholegrain cereals, legumes, eggs, dark green leafy vegetables, milk.

Vitamin	Benefits	Sources
Vitamin B6 (Pyridoxine)	Nervous system; skin, red blood cells.	Avocados, liver, peanuts, walnuts, pork, poultry, whole grains, egg yolks, lean meat, bananas, fish, potatoes.
Vitamin B12 (Cobalamin)	Healthy blood and nerves.	Liver, kidney, some fish (including shell fish), eggs, milk, milk products.
Vitamin C (Ascorbic acid)	Helps heal wounds, may fight colds, flu and infections; protects gums, keeps joints and ligaments in good working order.	Citrus fruits, potatoes, tomatoes, leafy greens
Biotin	Helps form fatty acids and release energy from carbohydrates and amino acids.	Liver, eggs, cereals, yeast
Folacin (Folic acid)	Helps form red blood cells and genetic material.	Liver, dark green leafy vegetables, orange juice, whole grain breads and cereals, enriched cereals, legumes

Chapter **12**

VALUABLE MINERALS

Like vitamins, a wide variety of minerals are essential for good health, growth and body functioning. Some, such as calcium and iron, are needed in quite large amounts, and for some people there is a real risk of deficiency if they do not eat a healthy diet.

Calcium – A regular supply of calcium is vital because bone tissue is constantly broken down and rebuilt. A calcium rich diet is particularly important during adolescence, pregnancy, breast-feeding, menopause, and for the elderly. Smoking, lack of exercise, too much alcohol, high protein and high salt intakes all encourage calcium losses.

Iron - Only a fraction of the iron present in food is absorbed, It is much more readily absorbed from red meat than from vegetable sources. Vitamin C also helps with absorption. Pregnant women, women who have heavy periods, and vegetarians should all be particularly careful about ensuring an adequate intake of iron.

Trace elements – These include other essential minerals such as zinc, iodine, magnesium, and potassium. Although important, they are only needed in minute quantities. They are found in a wide variety of foods and deficiency is very rare.

Mineral	Benefits	Sources
Calcium	Healthy bones, teeth and nails; muscle and nerve function, blood clotting; milk production in nursing mothers.	Cheese, milk, yoghurt, eggs, bread, nuts, pulses, fish with soft bones such as whitebait and tinned sardines, leafy green vegetables.

Mineral	Benefits	Sources
Chloride	Regulates fluid and electrolyte balances; forms part of gastric juice.	Salt, processed foods.
Magnesium	Needed for bone and teeth formation; aids in release of energy, nerve and muscle function.	Dark green leafy vegetables, nuts, seeds, whole grain foods, legumes, milk.
Phosphorus	Builds and strengthens bones; helps release energy from nutrients.	Milk, cheese, meat, fish, poultry, eggs, whole grains, legumes, nuts.
Potassium	Helps to transmit nerve impulses, control muscle contraction, and maintain proper blood pressure.	Many fruits and vegetables; cereals, legumes, and meat.
Sodium	Regulates fluid and acid base balance.	Salt, processed foods.
Sulphur	Needed to make hair, nails, and cartilage.	Meat, fish, eggs, and legumes.

Trace minerals are needed by the body in much smaller amounts, but are no less important for its functioning than the major minerals.

Mineral	Benefits	Sources
Chromium	Helps insulin work efficiently in glucose metabolism.	Brewer's yeast, calf's liver, whole-grain cereals, peanuts, wheat germ
Copper	Needed for iron absorption and metabolism; helps form red blood cells and nerve fibres	Liver, kidney, seafood, nuts, seeds, tap water.

Mineral	Benefits	Sources
Fluoride	Contributes to bone and teeth maintenance.	Fluoridated tap water, tea, and sardines with bones.
Iodine	Needed to form thyroid hormones.	Iodised salt, seafood, saltwater fish, dairy products, and vegetables.
Iron	Liver, red meat, oily fish, whole grain cereals, leafy green vegetables.	Makes haemoglobin, the pigment in red blood cells that helps transport oxygen around the body.
Manganese	Needed for bone formation, involved in fat synthesis.	Whole grains, fruits, vegetables, tea, legumes and nuts.
Molybdenum	Aids in metabolism	Milk, legumes, whole grain breads and cereals.
Selenium	Works in association with vitamin E as an antioxidant.	Liver, kidney, seafood, meat and whole sgrains.
Zinc	Needed for metabolism and digestion; aids in wound healing, growth, tissue repair, and sexual development.	Liver, seafood, meat, eggs, poultry, fish and whole grain cereals.

Fats and oils – are chemically similar compounds of carbon, hydrogen and oxygen, which are combined in a characteristic way to be different from one another. There are many different types of fats and oils. However, the only difference between fats and oil as a whole is that oils are liquid at room temperature. Most animal fats are hard at normal room temperature. Fats contain twice as much energy, weight for weight, as carbohydrates and so it is important to cut down on fats when dieting. However, fats and oils are important in cooking because they carry flavours and so they should be mixed judiciously with carbohydrate foods.

Fine Art of Balancing

A well balanced diet is the secret to being in good health and good shape. Balance is important to a healthy diet. The components of food that the body uses to sustain itself are known as nutrients. The nutrients in food fuel the body and provide the material needed for growth, for tissue maintenance and repair and for the regulation of physiological processes. When food is oxidised (burnt) in the body, the result is energy measured in kilocalories (the prefix "kilo" is usually dropped in non technical usage). Carbohydrates and fats are the body's main sources of energy, providing four and nine calories per gram respectively. Proteins also yield four calories per gram but is used as fuel only when energy from other sources is scarce. Vitamins and minerals are essential for body functioning, although they cannot be burnt as fuel. Strictly speaking, water and fibre are not nutrients, but water is vital to life and fibre plays an important role in elimination.

The human body has the ability to synthesise certain nutrients on its own. Those that it cannot make or cannot make in sufficient quantities (the vast majority) must be supplied by the foods you eat. Such nutrients are known as essential nutrients. If you don't get enough of them in your diet, you will develop potentially harmful deficiencies.

However no single type of food provides all the nutrients required for good health. You need to eat a wide variety of foods to got various nutrients.

Chapter **13**

FIBRE

What is Fibre?

Also known as roughage, fibre is a component of food that is more or less indigestible and can be found in all fruits, vegetables and whole grains. Fibres can be either insoluble (the less digestible bran fibre) or soluble (cellulose fibres from fruits and vegetables). For good health, you need both types of fibres in your diet.

Fibre is important to your body because it helps with the proper functioning of the intestinal tract as it speeds the elimination of waste products. It is a natural laxative and alleviates constipation. Those suffering from constipation should have a rich fibre diet. In addition, a rich fibre diet prevents against colon cancer, as there is less exposure of cancer causing agents to the intestinal tract.

Individuals with diabetes may also benefit from a high fibre diet since it modulates the rate at which glucose enters the blood and prevents increases in blood levels of sugar and insulin. Soluble fibre may also help to reduce cholesterol levels. Because fibre is filling, it provides a sense of satiety with far fewer calories than fat, thus controlling obesity and hypertension. A research done by the US-based Nurses Health Study found that the risk of heart attack was significantly lower among women who consumed an average of 23 grams of fibre.

Sources of Fibre

Whole grain bread and cereals; raw fruits and berries such as apples, plums, cherries, grapes, oranges, bananas, apricots, strawberries, raisins and dried fruits and vegetables such as beans, cabbage, carrot, cauliflower, celery cucumber, lettuce, onions and spinach. However, increase the fibre in your diet slowly to prevent abdominal bloating, gas and flatulence.

Importance of Fibre

Most of the foods we eat such as refined flour, polished rice, milk and milk products contain little fibre. Even vegetables have relatively little fibre. Fibre rich diets reduce blood sugar, serum cholesterol and relieve constipation, besides helping in prevention and treatment of several diseases such as colon cancer and cardiovascular diseases. For a healthy diet, one needs 20 to 35 gram of fibre, every day.

Five Great Tips to Fibre Up the System:

- **Change over to whole grains.** You consume a whole variety of cereals everyday but have you ever wondered whether it is whole grain or split or broken grain? Splitting means refining the cereal and as a result the grain loses a good part of the fibre. Try to change over to whole cereals in foods such as breads, pasta, flour, buns etc.
- **Eat legumes everyday.** Try and eat legumes daily, as they are one of the richest sources of fibre. Prefer whole pulses over split ones as they do not undergo much processing and hence are rich in nutrients.
- **Eat a minimum of five servings of fruits and vegetables every day.** Include vegetables in both lunch and dinner along with salads. This will take care of your four servings. Eat one or two fruits everyday and you can meet your five servings norm very easily.
- **Enjoy fruits and vegetables with edible peels.** This not only gives you fibre but also vital nutrients that are lost along with peels. Compare for yourself- a medium potato with peel has 3.6 grams of fibre whereas the fibre content of peeled potato reduces to 2.3. Also prefer whole fruits to juices, as juice is a refined form of fruit.
- **Eat a variety of foods.** Variety adds not only spice to your life but also good health. You end up consuming many different types of foods and hence take in a good number of nutrients, including fibre. Besides, you eat a well-balanced diet.

Fibre Facts

Certain foods like bread, rice, cereals, vegetables, fruit and nuts contain fibre. We should aim for 30 gms of fibre per day. Some of the good fibre sources are*–

Good Sources	Average Portion	Grams of Fibre
Wholemeal pasta	75 gms	9
Baked beans	125 gms	8
Frozen peas	75 gms	8
Bran flakes	50 gms	7
Banana	average fruit	3.5
Brown rice	50 gms	3
Cabbage	100 gms	3
Red kidney beans	40 gms	3
Wholemeal bread	1 large slice	3
High-fibre white bread	1 large slice	2

Chapter **14**

WATER

Not enough attention has been paid to water and its importance in diet. Water is necessary for our body to operate efficiently. Every cell in our body depends upon water to function properly. Most of us do not understand the role of this vital nutrient.

Up to 70 per cent of our total body weight comes from water. Inadequate intake of water could lead to major diseases that modern medicine can treat but fail to cure. Along with being a natural curative, a sip of water lowers body temperature, dilutes blood to the required consistency, promotes excretion of poisons from the skin in the form of evaporation, stimulates the normal functions of the kidneys and increases the movements of the intestines. Hot water works as a laxative and sedative and relieves pain, cramps and spasms. It also increases the metabolic rate and aids digestion.

Water acts as a solvent, coolant, lubricant and transport agent. The amount of body water varies with body fat. The percentage of water to body weight is greater in lean individuals. This is due to the nearly water free characteristics of fat tissue, which results in bodies with more fatty tissues containing proportionately less water than bodies with less fatty tissue.

Besides keeping body temperature stable, water carries nutrients, eliminates toxins and waste products, maintains blood volume and provides the medium in which chemical reactions occur in the cells.

The body has three sources of water: fluid intake, water content of food, and the fluid released during metabolism of proteins, carbohydrates and lipids.

Though thirst is the body's way of signalling that water is required, most of us ignore the signal. Most people, on average, drink only 3-4 glass of water per day as against the recommended intake of at least 6-8 glasses per day. The rest of the water the body needs must be extracted from other liquids or foods that we eat. Not enough water is a real threat to the system. Many chemical reactions inside the body will not occur without the right amount of water.

It only takes a one percent fluid loss in the body to become dehydrated.

This generally happens prior to any conscious sensation of being thirsty. Very small shortages of water can dramatically change and disrupt biochemistry. Exercise physiologists consider water as the single most important variable in peak performance. Your muscles can lose up to ten percent of their contractile strength and eight percent of speed from only three percent dehydration.

A small change makes a big difference when it comes to water. If you do a lot of travel by air, you can lose as much as two pounds of water in a three to four hour flight. Stress, alcohol and caffeine all influence the amount of water and the speed in which your body loses it. Any of these factors, alone or in combination, could cause a small but critical shrinkage of the brain. This small shrinkage will impair neuromuscular coordination, decrease concentration, and slow thinking. The average amount of water loss per day is two cups through breathing, two cups through invisible perspiration, and six cups through urination and bowel movements. That is a total of ten cups lost per day without taking into account perspiration from exercise or hard work, excessively dry air, alcohol or caffeine consumption.

Watery Facts

Blood is 83% water	55-65% of a woman's body is water
Muscles are 75% water	65-75% of a man's body is water
Bone is 22% water	An average adult body holds 35 to 50 litres of water.

Chapter **15**

ANTIOXIDANTS VS FREE RADICALS

In a perfect world, everything works together in harmony to create lush, productive, and beautiful landscapes. Energy is balanced and synergy abounds. The same idea applies to health when our bodies are fit and in chemical balance. But today's world is far from perfect. Our lives are typically stressful and we consume toxins on a daily basis, which ultimately alter our delicate biochemistry and wreak havoc on our trillions of internal chemical reactions. Compromised immune systems and increased exposure to free radicals eventually wear us down, age us prematurely, or bring on fearful diseases like cancer. But powerful natural compounds called antioxidants form a front line of defence that attack and neutralize the hordes of free radicals, helping us restore our health and live longer, happier lives.

A freshly cut apple will turn brown in a matter of minutes. Iron, when exposed to water and air, starts to rust. These chemical changes are the result of oxidation, the process by which a compound reacts with oxygen. Oxidation in the body creates free radicals in the fats, tissues, and bloodstream. The higher the number of free radicals, the greater the level of oxidative stress.

Oxygen is a critical element in the water we drink and the air that we breathe-without it we could not survive. Yet normal cellular reactions create toxic forms of oxygen that are free radicals such as super oxide, hydroxyl and lipid peroxides, singlet oxygen, and hydrogen peroxide. Small amounts of free radicals in the body are a good thing-too many, however, accelerate aging and disease.

Defining Free Radicals

Free radicals are atoms or molecules that contain at least one unpaired electron. To become electrically balanced, they steal electrons from other compounds in the body, which are usually critical parts of cells, tissue, or blood. These sites are injured, and the atom or molecule that loses its electron becomes a free radical itself, creating an unending chain reaction. Not all free radicals are bad. Free radicals produced by the immune system destroy viruses and bacteria. Others are involved in producing vital hormones and activating enzymes that are needed for life. But most of us are bombarded by a multitude of environmental toxins like smog, cigarette smoke, heavy metals, gasoline derivatives, ultraviolet radiation, and other carcinogenic chemicals that are also sources of free radicals. A healthy body can normally keep its free radicals in check, but if the immune system is weakened or the free radical load is too high, cellular damage results.

Bruce Ames, a research scientist at University of California-Berkeley, estimates that each cell in the human body suffers about 10,000 "hits" per day by free radicals. The extent of the damage is impressive: free radicals destroy enzymes, proteins, fat compounds, DNA molecules, and cell membranes and structures and alter the way cells code genetic material.

Free radical damage has a cumulative effect that interferes with cellular function, bogs down chemical reactions and neurological communications between cells, and speeds the growth of mutant cells and degenerative diseases like cancer, heart disease, and arthritis that are most common in older people. A significant cause of ageing is cellular free radical damage. As we get older, an increased amount of free radical garbage accumulates in our bodies. The good thing is that we are not completely powerless as antioxidant supplements can help protect us from the damage of free radical bombardment.

How Antioxidants Work

Antioxidants are compounds that neutralize free radicals by giving them the necessary electron they crave. Antioxidants can be vitamins, minerals, hormones, or enzymes. Although a certain amount is manufactured in the body as enzymes or hormones, most of our antioxidants come from fruits and vegetables.

Although many antioxidants can be obtained from food sources, it is difficult to get enough of them to hold back the free radicals constantly being generated in our polluted environment.

Certain antioxidants protect specific parts of the body against certain kinds of free radicals. For example, vitamin E protects the fats in cell membranes. Others such as ALA protect every cell in the body. In addition to fighting free radicals, antioxidants stimulate the immune system, reduce inflammation and fever, and help control pain. Once an antioxidant has neutralized a free radical, it is essentially "spent." Yet several antioxidants, including ALA and pycnogenol, can actually regenerate used vitamin C, which in turn reactivates used vitamin E.

Maintaining a healthy immune system, reducing stress, and consuming antioxidants can minimize free radical damage. Conditions that can be avoided or improved using antioxidant therapy include cancer, coronary heart disease, autoimmune disorders, rheumatoid arthritis, cataracts, diabetes, menopause, fertility, and neurological disorders such as Alzheimer's disease and Parkinson's disease.

Antioxidants Fight High Fat Meals

Researchers have measured how much damage just one high fat meal can cause. They've shown how, for at least six hours afterwards, arteries are unable to expand to properly handle the blood flow needed during physical or emotional stress. Scientists believe this may be one reason why people who already have "clogged" arteries so often suffer heart attacks soon after eating a high-fat meal. Scientists have suspected that a sudden high dose of fat triggers oxidation. This results in the release of certain chemicals in the body that damage the inner layer of cells that line the heart and blood vessels. They hypothesized that introducing antioxidants may counteract the process.

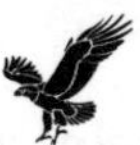

Chapter 16

CONSUME IN MODERATION

Eggs

Eggs are rich in protein, B vitamins, iron, and other minerals, all of which are essential for good health. But egg yolks are also rich in dietary cholesterol. An elevated cholesterol level in the blood is a major risk factor for coronary heart disease (which leads to heart attack). The American Heart Association recommends that healthy adults limit cholesterol intake to less than 300 milligrams (mg) per day. One large whole egg contains 213-220 mg of cholesterol. This is 71 percent of the daily-recommended amount.

This amount of cholesterol can be worked into eating plans in several ways. The key is not to focus on any one cholesterol-containing food. Instead, if a person chooses to get cholesterol in one form (e.g., by eating egg yolks), he or she must limit other dietary sources of cholesterol such as meat, poultry or dairy products.

Limiting the intake of egg yolks isn't hard. Many cholesterol-free egg substitutes and recipes that provide yolk-free alternatives are available.

Meat, Poultry and Fish

There was a time when meat was taken as the best food for health. Today, doctors recommend that red meat should be phased out of the diet and white meat should replace it. In any case, meat itself should be consumed in moderation.

Choose fish, shellfish, poultry (chicken and turkey) without the skin, and trimmed lean meats. Limit the intake of these to no more than 6 ounces (cooked), per day. Choose low-sodium, low-fat seasonings such as spices, herbs and other flavourings in cooking and at the table.

Select meat substitutes such as dried beans, peas, lentils or tofu (soybean curd).

Fish and Shellfish

Fish rank among the most nourishing of all foods. In fact, it is a good idea to replace all kinds of meat with fish. Fish contains about as much protein as meat. We know that eating fish helps lower cholesterol (the bad kind) and it is low in fat and calories so it can aid in weight loss if it's not fried or grilled in butter or oil. Now there's a new study that shows fish may help stave off certain types of cancers. A research study recently done in Milan, Italy compared 10,000 hospital patients who had cancer to 8,000 other patients who did not have cancer. Those who ate one or more servings a week showed a definite pattern of protection against cancers such as stomach, mouth, pharynx, oesophagus, colon and rectum. Fish may be an even healthier choice than previously thought. Recent studies have found that the omega oils contained in fish have beneficial effect on the heart.

Shrimp and crayfish are higher in cholesterol than most other types of fish, but lower in saturated fat and cholesterol than most meats and poultry.

Servings

A 3-ounce cooked portion is about the size of a deck of cards. To help you judge serving sizes, a 3-ounce portion equals:

- ❑ ½ of a chicken breast or a chicken leg with thigh (without skin)
- ❑ ¾ cup of flaked fish
- ❑ 2 thin slices of lean roast beef (each slice 3″ x 3″ x ¼″)
- ❑ Remove the skin and fat under the skin from poultry pieces before cooking (except when roasting a whole chicken or turkey - remove the skin before carving and serving the meat). Select whole turkeys that haven't been injected with fats or broths.
- ❑ Choose cuts of meat that have the least amount of visible fat and trim this visible fat off meat.

- Instead of frying, prepare meat by baking, broiling, roasting, micro waving or stir-frying. Pour off the fat after browning. Chill meat juices after cooking, so that you can easily skim off the hardened fat. Then you can add the meat to stews, soups and gravy. Organ meats are very high in cholesterol. However, liver is rich in iron and vitamins and a small serving (3 ounces) is OK about once a month.

Sugar

Here is some bad news for the sweet toothed. Excess of sugar is detrimental to health. When eaten in moderation as part of a balanced diet, sugar provides pleasure for the palate. On the negative side, however, sugar not only promotes tooth decay, but when it is eaten in excess, the empty calories that sugar supplies can take the place of important nutrients in the diet.

Here are some tips on how to cut on sugar intake –

- Educate yourself about which foods contain large amounts of sugar and eat less of them either by having them less often or by eating smaller portions.
- Read food labels carefully to find hidden sources of sugar. Avoid foods that list a sugar first or list a variety of different calorific sweeteners such as corn syrup or fructose.
- Choose unsweetened breakfast cereals and eat them with fresh fruit rather than sugar.
- Eliminate or cut back on sugared soft drinks. Substitute club soda, unsweetened juices or plain water.
- Serve fresh fruit or fruit packed in its own juice instead of dried fruit or canned fruit packed in syrup, which are both much higher in sugar.
- Save pastries and rich cakes for occasional treats only.
- Prepare sauces, puddings, cookies, cakes, pies, and other potentially sugary foods from starch instead of buying commercial varieties or using mixes. In many cases, you can significantly reduce the amount of sugar and other caloric sweeteners in such food without compromising on taste or texture. Experiment with spices and herbs

such as vanilla, cinnamon, nutmeg and ginger to retain flavour without adding lots of extra calories. Instead of frosting a cake, sprinkle a little powdered sugar on it.

- ❑ Gradually reduce the amount of sugar or honey that you put in coffee or tea.
- ❑ Don't keep candy and sweets around the house to nibble on.
- ❑ Don't reward children with sweets, and ask friends and relatives to respect your policy.

Caffeine

For long coffee and tea have been seen as a necessity of life, but the recent discoveries indicate that too much of caffeine could be counter-productive. Moderation is the watchword for caffeine consumption.

Caffeine is a central nervous system stimulant found in more than 60 plants, with coffee beans, cocoa beans, tealeaves, and the kola nut being the major dietary sources. In addition to occurring naturally in coffee, tea, cocoa and chocolate, caffeine is added to many soft drinks and over-the -counter and prescription preparations.

Caffeine is absorbed quickly and distributed throughout the body, reaching peak levels in the blood within 15-45 minutes. In most people, it increases alertness and reduces fatigue. Scientists believe that caffeine works by blocking adenosine, a compound that, in the brain, acts as a brake on stimulants. Caffeine perks you up by reversing the effects of adenosine.

In people who are sensitive to it or ingest a lot of it, caffeine can cause restlessness, anxiety, jitters, tremors, sleep disturbances, headaches, a temporary rise in blood pressure, rapid or irregular heartbeat, increased production of urine, upset stomach, or other unpleasant symptoms. Recent studies also suggest that caffeine could rob the addicts of bone density. Most people develop a tolerance to caffeine. Someone who normally doesn't take caffeine may become anxious and jittery after a single cup of coffee, while a person used to drinking six mugs may feel no adverse effects. The current average daily level of caffeine consumption is about 200 milligrams (2-3 cups of coffee, depending on the brewing method). A single cup of Indian coffee contains up to 100 milligrams of caffeine.

Judge your own caffeine tolerance by its impact on you. Coffee is addictive and habit forming. If you drink coffee or colas and are restless, anxious, and shaky or have trouble falling asleep, it may be time to cut back on caffeine or eliminate it altogether. Reduce your intake gradually over a week or two to avoid withdrawal symptoms, such as headaches, lethargy, and drowsiness.

Decaffeinated coffee - decaffeinated coffee does not contain chemical residues in appreciable amounts.

Caffeine Levels

The caffeine content of a cup of coffee depends on the type of bean and how it was processed and brewed. Tea's caffeine content increases the longer it steeps.

Item **Caffeine (mg)**	**Coffee (1 cup)**
Regular, drip	60-180
Regular, percolated	40-170
Regular, instant	30-120
Decaffeinated, brewed	2-5
Decaffeinated, instant	1-5
Tea (1 Cup)	
Brewed	25-110
Instant	25-50
Cola drinks and chocolate	
Cola drinks (1 bottle)	30-60
Chocolate milk (250 ml)	2-7
Cocoa (1 cup)	2-20

Sodium

Common table salt, known chemically as sodium chloride, is the main source of sodium in our diets. Sodium is an essential nutrient required by the body to help regulate its fluid balance, maintain heart rhythm, conduct nerve impulses, and contract muscles. For body requirement, a safe minimum is 500 milligrams of sodium, about a quarter teaspoon of table salt is enough. Most people consume about twice the daily maximum (3000 milligram of sodium - about teaspoon and a half of table salt) recommended by doctors.

Reduction of sodium intake to 1 millimole per kilogram of ideal body weight will lower blood pressure in those with hypertension. In others, it will prevent hypertension from too much sodium. If sodium intake is reduced while people are young, the rise in blood pressure with age could be prevented.

The relationship between salt intake and hypertension (high blood pressure) is complex and not fully understood but the direct relationship between sodium consumption and the high incidence of high blood pressure has been demonstrated in a number of studies. About 10-15 percent of people are actually 'sodium-sensitive'; meaning that consuming too much salt directly elevates their blood pressure.

Healthy adults should reduce their sodium intake to not more than 2400 milligrams per day. This is about 1¼ teaspoons of sodium chloride (salt). To illustrate, the following are sources of sodium in the diet.

¼ teaspoon salt = 500 mg sodium
½ teaspoon salt = 1000 mg sodium
¾ teaspoon salt = 1500 mg sodium
1 teaspoon salt = 2000 mg sodium
1 teaspoon baking soda = 1000 mg sodium

Where is the sodium in the foods we eat?

There are two major sources of sodium in the foods we eat. It is present in raw foods but the major source is sodium, which is added. This occurs during manufacture and preparation of food. Additional amounts in the forms of sodium chloride may be in sauces and flavouring agents.

What is a normal sodium requirement?

The amount of sodium required will depend on ideal body weight and is equivalent to 1 mmol per kilogram, per day. A man who, for example, is 176 cm tall and weighs 70 kg possesses ideal body weight. Therefore, his recommended dietary sodium intake is 70 mmol of sodium per day. Ten mmols (millimoles) or meq (milli-equivalents) of sodium is contained in 0.58 grams of sodium chloride. Sodium makes up 40% of sodium chloride by weight.

Infants require less sodium (10-49 mmols a day) than adults. Sufficient sodium to meet baby's needs is present in breast milk even though, when compared with cow's milk, breast milk has only one-third amount of sodium. Older children up to their teens will need a slightly higher sodium intake per body weight than adults.

Sources of salt

There are many hidden sources of salt. One of the main sources of sodium in the diet is the group of staple items – bread, butter or margarine and cheese. Breads generally contain salt and so do biscuits. Cheese is very high in salt. Apart from these most of the processed foods like gravy powder, stock cubes, yeast extracts, peanut butter, pickles and olives also contain sodium.

Some minor sources of sodium in our diet are mineral replacement drinks, mega doses of vitamin C and some soluble painkillers.

The natural sodium content of fresh foods does not really present a problem because it is relatively low in most foods. Some seafoods are among the exception. Prawns and scallops, for example, have significant sodium content but these do not usually form a large part of most people's diet.

Protein foods from animal sources also have a relatively high content of sodium but, as the healthy diet pyramid indicates, we should all decrease our intake of animal products.

Milk, being an animal protein product, falls into this group and the recommended intake for an adult is 300 ml and, generally, this should not be exceeded.

Fruits and vegetables contain insignificant amounts of sodium and are abundant sources of potassium fibre and vitamins. Increasing the potassium content of the diet is thought to have a beneficial effect on blood pressure, so it is recommended that consumption of fruit and vegetables be increased.

It is true that some vegetables, like spinach and silver beet, contain significant amounts of sodium. However, they also have a very high content of potassium and their sodium content is much lower than most processed foods. It is wise to have at least three servings of vegetables and three of fruits daily. The best snacks and desserts are fresh fruit.

High sodium items

- All canned, corned, and pickled meat or salted meat or fish. All processed meat e.g. corned beef, salami, chicken loaf, ham, bacon, sausages, frankfurter, tinned fish unless labelled no added salt.
- All hard cheese, especially Parmesan or Romano. Highly salted breakfast cereals, commercial cakes, pastries, buns, cake mixes. Take care with commercial dry biscuits and sweet biscuits, which can contain significant amounts of sodium.
- All canned vegetables unless labelled no added salt. Pickles, sauerkraut, minted frozen peas.
- All takeaway foods.
- All canned and packet soups, prepared sauces or sauce mixes, gravy powders, stock cubes, meat extracts, yeast extracts, vegetable salts, celery salt, garlic salt, lemon pepper, monosodium glutamate, commercial mayonnaise or salad dressings, commercial sauces, soya sauce, olives, salted nuts, snack foods e.g., potato crisps, meat and fish pastes, ordinary peanut butter.
- Milk chocolate, caramels, Dutch liquorice, fizzy lollies.

Fats

Fats in themselves are not harmful; it's the high fat diet typical of many countries that can cause problems. Dietary fat is the body's most concentrated source of energy, supplying more than twice as many calories per gram (9) as carbohydrates (4). Most of the fats in food are triglycerides, combinations of three fatty acids and glycerol (an oily alcohol); in addition, animal foods contain small amounts of fatlike substance called cholesterol. Triglycerides are broken down in the small intestine into glycerol and fatty acids. As fatty acids are absorbed from the intestine via the lymphatic system into the bloodstream, they facilitate the absorption of the fat-soluble vitamins A, D, E, and K. in addition, fatty acids from certain polyunsaturated fats are required for the growth and maintenance of body tissues and other vital functions.

Beside, from its nutritional importance, fat enhances the texture and flavour of foods and creates a pleasant feeling of fullness. In other words, people like fat and tend to eat too much of it. To maintain good health, however, you need only about 1 tablespoon of polyunsaturated fat a day and you don't need any saturated or monounsaturated fat. Unfortunately, most people consume much more than a tablespoon of fat a day, a habit that can have serious health consequences.

Protein, carbohydrates, and fat can be converted into body fat, which is simply the form in which the body stores excess energy. But since dietary fat is such a concentrated source of energy, it is potentially the most fattening of all the macronutrients. Dietary fat has also been implicated in two of our deadliest diseases: cancer and heart disease. Diets high in total fat have been linked with an increased risk of cancer of the colon, rectum, breast, or prostate, while diets high in saturated fat are associated with high levels of blood cholesterol, clogged arteries, and coronary heart disease.

There are three kinds of fats in the foods we eat:

- ❑ Saturated – come mainly from animal products (milk, butter, cheese, and meat) and in excess is thought to contribute to raise cholesterol levels.

- ❑ Polyunsaturated – are found in vegetable oils such as sunflower, safflower, corn and soya bean oils; they are also found in some fish oils and some nuts, and are said to help lower cholesterol levels.
- ❑ Monounsaturated fatty acids – are found in olive and rapeseed oils; they are also said to lower cholesterol levels.

Most foods contain all three types of fat, but in varying amounts. Only saturated fats and dietary cholesterol raise blood cholesterol. A high level of cholesterol in the blood is a major risk factor for coronary heart disease, which leads to heart attack.

The body can use all three types of fats, but doctors recommend that an average person should limit total fat intake (saturated, monounsaturated, polyunsaturated) to no more than 30 percent of total calories.

Saturated fat intake should be limited to 7-10 percent of total calories each day.

- ❑ Polyunsaturated fat calories should be up to 10 percent of total calories.
- ❑ Monounsaturated fat intake should be up to 15 percent of total calories.

What are saturated fatty acids?

Saturated fats are usually solid at room temperature, and they're more stable - that is, they don't combine readily with oxygen. Saturated fatty acids have all the hydrogen the carbon atoms can hold. Saturated fat is the main dietary factor in raising blood cholesterol. The main sources of saturated fat are foods from animals and some plants.

Cholesterol Facts

A white, waxy, fatlike substance, cholesterol is a naturally occurring component of cell membranes and nerve sheaths. It also plays a role in the manufacture of bile acids, steroid hormones, and vitamin D, and it helps transport fats in the bloodstream. In our body, the liver makes most of the cholesterol in the blood. Whatever its source, cholesterol journeys through the bloodstream as part of 'packages' called lipoproteins that also contain protein and triglyceride, the main form of body fat.

You get cholesterol in two ways. Your body makes some of it, and the rest comes from animal products that you eat, such as meats, poultry, fish, eggs, butter, cheese and whole milk. Food from plants like fruits, vegetables and cereals do not have cholesterol. Cholesterol and other fats can't dissolve in the blood. They have to be transported to and from the cells by special carriers called lipoproteins and there are two kinds that you need to be concerned with. Low-density lipoprotein, or LDL, is known as the "bad" cholesterol. Too much LDL cholesterol can clog the arteries to your heart and increase your risk of heart attack. High-density lipoprotein, or HDL, is known as the "good" cholesterol. Your body makes HDL cholesterol for your protection. It travels away from your arteries. Studies suggest that high levels of HDL cholesterol reduce your risk of heart attack.

High density lipoproteins (HDL)

High-density lipoproteins (HDL): the "good" cholesterol. HDL carries cholesterol in the blood from other parts of the body back to the liver, which leads to its removal from the body. So HDL helps keep cholesterol from building up in the walls of the arteries.

HDL-cholesterol levels

Less than 35 mg/dL is a major risk factor for heart disease
35 to 59 mg/dL is considered normal but the higher your HDL, the better.
An HDL of 60 mg/dL and above is considered protective against heart disease

Note: These categories apply to adults age 20 and above.

Low density lipoproteins (LDL)

What is LDL cholesterol?

Low-density lipoprotein is the major cholesterol carrier in the blood. If too much LDL cholesterol circulates in the blood, it can slowly build up in the walls of the arteries feeding the heart and brain. Together with other substances it can form plaque, a thick, hard deposit that can clog those arteries. This condition is known as arteriosclerosis. A clot (thrombus) that forms in the region of this plaque can block the flow of blood to part of the heart muscle and cause a heart attack. If a clot blocks the flow of blood to part of the brain, the result is a stroke. A high level of LDL cholesterol (more than 130 mg/dL) reflects an increased risk of heart disease. That's why LDL cholesterol is often called "bad" cholesterol. Lower levels of LDL cholesterol reflect a lower risk of heart disease

LDL-cholesterol levels

Less than 130 mg/dL-Desirable
130 to 159 mg/dL Borderline-High Risk
160 mg/dL and above-High Risk

Note: These categories apply to adults age 20 and above.

Why is LDL cholesterol considered bad?

A high level (more than 160 mg/dL or higher than 130 mg/dL if you have two or more risk factors for cardiovascular disease) of low-density lipoprotein, or LDL cholesterol, reflects an increased risk of heart disease. That's why LDL cholesterol is often called "bad" cholesterol. Lower levels of LDL cholesterol reflect a lower risk of heart disease.

Why is HDL cholesterol considered "good"?

About one-third to one-fourth of blood cholesterol is carried by high-density lipoprotein (HDL). HDL cholesterol is known as the "good" cholesterol because a high level of HDL cholesterol seems to protect against heart attack. Medical experts think that HDL tends to carry cholesterol away from the arteries and back to the liver, where it is passed from the body. Low HDL cholesterol levels (lower than 35 mg/dL) may result in a greater risk for heart disease.

Fats that raise cholesterol

- **Dietary cholesterol** - found in foods from animals e.g. meats, egg yolks, dairy products, organ meats, fish and poultry

- **Saturated fats** – found in foods from animals e.g. whole milk, cream, ice cream, whole-milk cheeses, butter, lard and meats.
- **Certain plant oils** like palm, palm kernel and coconut oils, cocoa butter also contain this type of cholesterol.

Fats that lower cholesterol

- Polyunsaturated fats - can be obtained from certain plant oils like safflower, sesame, soy, corn and Sunflower-seed oils, nuts and seeds
- Monounsaturated fats – found in certain plant oils, olive, canola and peanut oils, avocados.

What about hydrogenated fats?

During food processing, fats may undergo a chemical process known as hydrogenation. Hydrogenation means to add hydrogen, or, in the case of fatty acids, to saturate. The process changes liquid oil, naturally high in unsaturated fatty acids, to a more solid and more saturated form. The greater the degree of hydrogenation, the more saturated the fat becomes. Many commercial products contain hydrogenated or partially hydrogenated vegetable oils.

Recent studies suggest that these fats may raise blood cholesterol. Hydrogenated fats in margarine and other fats are acceptable if the product contains liquid vegetable oil as the first ingredient and no more than 2 grams of saturated fat per tablespoon. The fatty acid content of most margarines and spreads is printed on the package or label.

What are polyunsaturated and monounsaturated fatty acids?

Polyunsaturated and monounsaturated fatty acids make up the total of unsaturated fatty acids. Unsaturated fats have at least one unsaturated bond - that is, at least one place that hydrogen can be added to the molecule. They're often found in liquid oils of vegetable origin.

Polyunsaturated oils are liquid at room temperature and in the refrigerator. They easily combine with oxygen in the air to become rancid. Monounsaturated oils are liquid at room temperature but start to solidify at refrigerator temperatures.

Polyunsaturated fats tend to help the body get rid of newly formed cholesterol. Thus, they keep the blood cholesterol level down and reduce cholesterol deposits in artery walls. Recent research has shown that monounsaturated fats may also help reduce blood cholesterol as long as the diet is very low in saturated fat. Both types of unsaturated fats may help lower your blood cholesterol level when used in place of saturated fats in your diet. But you should be moderate in your intake of all types of fat.

Poly or monounsaturated oils - and margarines and spreads made from these oils - should be used in limited amounts. Choose fats and oils that contain less than 2 grams of saturated fat per tablespoon.

Oils – oils are chemically similar to fats; the difference is simply that oils are liquid at room temperature whereas fats are solid.

Cooking with Oils

Corn oil – although corn oil is healthy, this is the least satisfactory of the recommended vegetable oils for cooking purposes. For salads, the flavour is rather powerful. If you do not find the flavour attractive, try mixing in some olive oil for cooking or salads.

Olive oil – Olive oil is delicious for everything, but is expensive. It has a lovely fruity flavour, which varies tremendously from country to country. However, it is wasteful to use this oil for frying, since it loses its delicious flavour at high temperatures. Use it for rubbing on to meat or fish before grilling, for marinades, for lubricating freshly cooked pasta, and of course for all salads.

Salad oil – mixing four tablespoons of sunflower oil with two dessertspoons of walnut oil, which has a delicious flavour, can make an interesting salad oil.

Soya oil – good oil for frying, but it starts to taste and smell a bit strong at high temperatures. It has the right consistency for salads. This is the oil used in Japan, where they have so little heart disease. Nutritionally, it is a highly recommended oil.

Sunflower oil – the sunflower oil is excellent for frying as it is almost tasteless and does not smell. It gives a very crisp result. As it is so light and thin it makes a rather dull salad dressing. It is the most versatile of the recommended polyunsaturated oils but it is expensive.

Composition of fats and oils – Fats and oils high in polyunsaturated and mono-unsaturated constituents are the best for health.

Item	Saturated	Mono-unsaturated	Poly-unsaturated
Beef	48%	44%	3%
Chicken	32%	37%	26%
Lamb	54%	37%	4%
Pork	36%	42%	17%
Liver	34%	27%	34%
Herring	19%	10%	66%
Milk, butter, cheddar	62%	30%	3%
Eggs	33%	45%	17%
Vegetable oils			
Coconut	91%	7%	2%
Corn	17.5%	29%	56.5%
Ground nut	13%	61%	24%
Olive	11%	74%	10%
Palm	53%	38%	9%
Safflower	11.5%	13%	75.5%
Soya bean	17%	25%	58%
Sunflower	12%	20%	68%

16 simple ways to reduce fat in diet

- ❑ Reduce serving sizes to 25-28 gms (about the size of a deck of cards), and do not eat seconds. If you like red meat, choose the leanest cuts, such as tenderloin, flank steak, chuck top and bottom round, or lean veal. Eat more poultry and fish. They contain less saturated fat than red meat.
- ❑ Remove all visible fat before cooking. Poultry skin may be removed either before or after cooking. Broil or bake instead of frying. Replace some meat proteins with a combination of legumes (dried beans, peas, lentils) and grains. Use skim, ½, or I percent milk. Choose cheeses made with skim or part skim milk, or look for cheeses that have no more than five grams of fat per ounce (read the label).
- ❑ Try low-fat or non-fat cottage cheese or yoghurt in place of cream and sour cream, or use fat-free sour cream and Cream cheese.
- ❑ Steam vegetables. If you choose to sauté them, use one tablespoon of oil (or less), or try using other liquids such as wine, defatted broth, or cooking sherry. Use non-stick pans, or add oil to a preheated pan (less oil goes further this way).
- ❑ Season vegetables with herbs and spices instead of butter and sauces, or try butter substitutes.
- ❑ Experiment with using less oil than is called for in recipes. Avoid high-fat crackers, chips, non-dairy creamers, and margarines made with hydrogenated oil, palm oil, coconut oil, or cocoa butter.
- ❑ Eat plenty of carbohydrates to fill you up (fruits, vegetables, grains, bread, pasta, etc.). Let salads go naked, or eat them modestly dressed in lemon juice or fat-free mayonnaise or dressing. Use fresh vegetable and tomato sauces instead of rich cream sauces on pasta.

Triglyceride connection

Triglyceride is a form of fat. It comes from food and is also made in your body. People with high triglycerides often have high total cholesterol, high LDL cholesterol and a low HDL cholesterol level. Many people with heart disease also have high triglyceride levels. Several clinical studies have shown that people with above-normal triglyceride levels (greater than or equal to 200 mg/dL) have an increased risk of heart disease. People with diabetes or who are obese are also likely to have high triglycerides.

What about cholesterol and diet?

People get cholesterol in two ways. The body - mainly the liver - produces varying amounts, usually about 1,000 milligrams a day. Another 400 to 500 mg (or more) can come directly from foods. Foods from animals (especially egg yolks, meat, poultry, fish, seafood and whole-milk dairy products) contain cholesterol. Foods from plants (fruits, vegetables, grains, nuts and seeds) don't contain cholesterol. Typically the body makes all the cholesterol it needs, so people don't need to consume it.

Saturated fatty acids are the chief culprit in raising blood cholesterol, which increases your risk of heart disease. But dietary cholesterol also plays a part. The average man consumes about 337 milligrams of cholesterol a day; the average woman, 217 milligrams. Some of the excess dietary cholesterol is removed from the body through the liver. Still, the doctors and nutritionists recommend that you limit your average daily cholesterol intake to less than 300 milligrams. If you have heart disease, limit your daily intake to less than 200 milligrams. Still, everyone should remember that by keeping their dietary intake of saturated fats low, they would also be able to significantly lower their dietary cholesterol intake.

Foods high in saturated fat generally contain substantial amounts of dietary cholesterol. People with severe hyper cholesterolemia may need an even greater reduction. Since cholesterol is present in all foods from animal sources, care must be taken to eat no more than six ounces of lean meat, fish and poultry per day and to use skim (fat-free) and low-fat dairy products. High-quality proteins from vegetable source such as beans are good substitutes for animal sources of protein.

How does exercise (physical activity) affect cholesterol?

For some people, exercise affects blood cholesterol level by increasing HDL ("good") cholesterol. Higher HDL cholesterol is linked with decreased risk of heart disease. Exercise can also help control weight, diabetes, and high blood pressure. Exercise that uses oxygen to provide energy to large muscles (aerobic exercise) raises your heart and breathing rates. Regular exercise such as brisk walking, jogging and swimming also condition your heart and lungs. Physical inactivity has been established as a major risk factor for heart disease. Even moderate-intensity activities, if done daily, help reduce your risk. Examples are walking for pleasure, gardening, housework, dancing and yoga.

How does cigarette / tobacco affect cholesterol?

Cigarette and tobacco smoke is one of the six major risk factors of heart disease that you can change, treat or modify. Smoking has been shown to lower HDL ("good") cholesterol levels.

How does alcohol affect cholesterol?

In some studies, moderate use of alcohol is linked with higher HDL ("good") cholesterol levels. However, the benefit isn't great enough to recommend drinking alcohol if you don't do so already. If you drink, do so in moderation. Incidence of heart disease in those who consume moderate amounts of alcohol (an average of one to two drinks per day for men and one drink per day for women) is lower than in non-drinkers.

However, with increased consumption of alcohol, there are other health dangers, such as alcoholism, high blood pressure, obesity, stroke, cancer, etc.

Lowering cholesterol

Genes and diet both influence cholesterol levels. You can't alter your genetic heritage, but in most cases, a diet low in saturated fat and cholesterol will help keep your blood cholesterol levels down. Although eating too much cholesterol rich food does raise blood cholesterol levels, the main culprit is saturated fat. The specifics of a cholesterol-lowering diet vary, but in general you should restrict fat intake to less than 30% of your total daily calories; saturated fat to less than 10% of total calories; polyunsaturated fat, to no more than 10% of total calories; and cholesterol, to less than 300 mg per day.

If your blood cholesterol levels are very high or if dieting does not lead to improvement within three months, your doctor may suggest a further reduction in your saturated fat intake to less than 7% of your total calories, and in your cholesterol intake to less than 200 mg per day. If this more restrictive diet fails to lower your blood cholesterol levels after 3-6 months, a cholesterol-lowering drug may also be prescribed. Although such drugs are effective, people taking them still have to stick to their diet.

Whatever it takes, bringing down high cholesterol levels is well worth the effort. Every 1%decrease in blood cholesterol results in a 2% drop in heart disease risk. Even if your blood cholesterol levels are not evaluated, following a diet low in saturated fats and cholesterol is still in the best interest of your heart and your general health.

What makes cholesterol high or low?

Your blood cholesterol level is affected not only by what you eat but also by how quickly your body makes LDL ("bad") cholesterol and disposes of it. In fact, your body makes all the cholesterol it needs, and it is not necessary to take in any additional cholesterol from the foods you eat. Many factors help determine whether your LDL-cholesterol level is high or low.

The following factors are the most important:

- Heredity
- What you eat
- Weight
- Physical activity/exercise
- Age and sex
- Alcohol
- Stress

Heredity: Your genes influence how high your LDL ("bad") cholesterol by affecting how fast LDL is made and removed from the blood. One specific form of inherited high cholesterol that affects 1 in 500 people is familial hyper cholesterolemia, which often leads to early heart disease. But even if you do not have a specific genetic form of high cholesterol, genes play a role in influencing your LDL-cholesterol level.

What you eat: Two main nutrients in the foods you eat make your LDL ("bad") cholesterol level go up: saturated fat, a type of fat found mostly in foods that come from animals; and cholesterol, which comes only from animal products. Saturated fat raises your LDL-cholesterol level more than anything else in the diet. Eating too much saturated fat and cholesterol is the main reason for high levels of cholesterol and a high rate of heart attacks. Reducing the amount of saturated fat and cholesterol you eat is a very important step in reducing your blood cholesterol levels.

Weight: Excess weight tends to increase your LDL ("bad") cholesterol level. If you are overweight and have a high LDL-cholesterol level, losing weight may help you lower it. Weight loss also helps to lower triglycerides and raise HDL ("good") cholesterol levels.

Physical activity/exercise: Regular physical activity may lower LDL ("bad") cholesterol and raise HDL ("good") cholesterol levels.

Age and sex: Before menopause, women usually have total cholesterol levels that are lower than those of men of the same age. As women and men get older, their blood cholesterol levels rise until about 60 to 65 years of age. In women, menopause often causes an increase in their LDL ("bad") cholesterol and a decrease in their HDL ("good") cholesterol level, and after the age of 50, women often have higher total cholesterol levels than men of the same age.

Alcohol: Alcohol intake increases HDL ("good") cholesterol but does not lower LDL ("bad") cholesterol. Doctors don't know for certain whether alcohol also reduces the risk of heart disease. Drinking too much alcohol can damage the liver and heart muscle, lead to high blood pressure, and raise triglycerides. Because of the risks, alcoholic beverages should not be used as a way to prevent heart disease.

Stress: Stress over the long term has been shown in several studies to raise blood cholesterol levels. One way that stress may do this is by affecting your habits. For example, when some people are under stress, they console themselves by eating fatty foods. The saturated fat and cholesterol in these foods contribute to higher levels of blood cholesterol.

Controlling your fat intake

To keep calories derived from fat fewer than 30% of your daily calorie total (and saturated fats and polyunsaturated fats each under 10%) may require changes in how you eat, shop and cook. Follow these tips for reducing the fat content of your diet –

- ❑ Eat lean meats and poultry
- ❑ Don't fry or sauté foods in fat; use a non-stick pan with broth or try baking, broiling, poaching, roasting, or steaming instead.
- ❑ If you do cook or season foods with oil, choose among those oils that are lowest in saturated fat. Avoid palm and coconut oil, which are highly saturated.
- ❑ Cook meat, fish or poultry on a rack so that fat drips away; baste with fat-free wine, fruit juices, or broth. Don't serve drippings.
- ❑ Trim fat from meat and trim skin and fat from poultry before cooking.
- ❑ Cook stews and soups ahead of time and chill. Remove the congealed fat and reheat.
- ❑ Cut down on peanut butter, avocadoes, coconut meat, and olives.
- ❑ Read food labels carefully, avoid foods with high levels of fat, particularly saturated or hydrogenated fats.
- ❑ Cut down on high-fat snacks such as buttered popcorn, chips, cookies, pastries, chocolate candy and cakes. If you must nibble, try raw vegetables, air-popped popcorn, or fresh fruit.

- Try low-fat or fat-free versions of normally high-fat foods like salad dressings, sour cream, mayonnaise and whipped cream.
- Go for fruit ices, which have no fat, instead of ice creams, which have a great deal of fat.

Calculating your daily fat quotas and interpreting the fat content information found of food labels can be difficult.

Two Useful Formulas

- To figure the maximum number of calories you should derive from fat per day, multiply your total daily calorie intake by 30% (0.3); divide the result by 9 (calories per gram of fat) for your maximum daily quota of fat in grams. A third of this figure is your limit for saturated fats and for polyunsaturated fats. An active man who consumes 2,800 calories a day should restrict his daily fat intake to under 840 fat calories (2,800x0.3), or 93 grams of fat (840/9). His intake of saturated fat and polyunsaturated fat should not exceed 280 calories (31 grams) each.
- To figure the percentage of fat calories in a food, multiply the grams of fat in a serving by 9 and then divide the result by the total calories per serving. For example, a cup of whole milk contains 9 grams of fat and 150 calories, 48% of which come from fat (8x9÷ 150=0.48).

Table For Diets at Three-Calorie Levels

Calories Required	Cereals Group (Servings)	Vegetables Group (Servings)	Fruit Group (Servings)	Milk Group (Servings)	Meat Group (Grams)	Fat and Oils (Grams)
1600 Calories (Lower)	6	3	2	2-3	145	53
2200 Calories (Moderate)	9	4	3	2-3	175	73
2800 Calories (Higher)	11	5	4	2-3	200	93

Total added sugar for 1600 calories – 6 teaspoons
For 2200 calories – 12 teaspoons
For 2800 calories – 18 teaspoons

Servings

1 slice of bread = 1 serving
1 cup rice = 2 servings
1 cup raw leafy vegetables = 1 serving
1 medium apple, banana, orange
1/2 cup of chopped, cooked, or canned fruit
3/4 cup of fruit juice, Milk, Yoghurt, and Cheese
1 cup of milk or yoghurt

This is just a basic grid; work out the details in consultation with your dietician or doctor.

The next time you say that you are putting on weight without eating too much, just do the calorie counting and you will know what is wrong with your diet.

Some Good, Some Bad

By now everyone is aware that food can broadly be divided into two types – the good and the bad in the sense that the good ones are good for our body while the intake of the bad foods should be controlled because they can be harmful. The good elements are friends of our body.

Chapter **17**

VEGETARIAN FOODS

What is a "Vegetarian" Food?

Some people choose to follow a "vegetarian" diet, but there is no single vegetarian-eating pattern. The vegan or total vegetarian diet is only foods of plant origin: fruits, vegetables, legumes (dried beans and peas), grains, seeds and nuts. The lacto-vegetarian diet is plant foods plus cheese and other dairy products. The ovo-lacto-vegetarian (or lacto-ovo-vegetarian) diet also includes eggs.

Are Vegetarian Diets Healthy?

Since vegetarian diets are low in animal products, they are typically lower than nonvegetarian diets in total fat, saturated fat, and cholesterol. These factors are associated with increased risk of obesity, coronary heart disease (which causes heart attack), high blood pressure, diabetes mellitus, and some forms of cancer. Thus, it is logical that vegetarian diets are healthful and nutritionally adequate when appropriately planned.

Nutrients in Vegetarian Foods

Protein: You don't need to eat animal products to have enough protein in your diet. Plant proteins alone can provide enough of the essential and non-essential amino acids, as long as sources of dietary protein are varied and caloric intake is high enough to meet energy needs. Whole grains, legumes, vegetables, seeds and nuts all contain both essential and non-essential amino acids. Soya protein has been shown to be equal to proteins of animal origin. It can be the sole protein source if desired.

Iron: Vegetarians may have a greater risk of iron deficiency than non-vegetarians. The richest sources of iron are red meat, liver and egg yolk - all high in cholesterol. Dried beans, spinach, enriched products; brewer's yeast and dried fruits are all good plant sources of iron.

Vitamin B-12: Comes naturally from animal sources only. Vegans need a reliable source of vitamin B-12, which can be found in some fortified (not enriched) breakfast cereals, fortified soya beverages, some brands of nutritional (brewer's) yeast and other foods (check the labels), as well as vitamin supplements.

Vitamin D: Vegans should have a reliable source of vitamin D. A supplement may be needed for vegans who get little sunlight. Calcium: Studies have shown that vegetarians absorb and retain more calcium from foods than do non-vegetarians. Vegetable greens such as spinach, kale and broccoli, and some legumes and soybean products are good sources of calcium from plants.

Zinc: Zinc is needed for growth and development. Good plant sources include grains, nuts and legumes. Care should be taken in selecting supplements containing no more than 15-18 mg zinc because supplements containing 50 mg or more may lower HDL ("good") cholesterol in some people.

Tips for vegetarians

- ❑ Vegetarian diets of any type should include a wide variety of foods and enough calories to meet your energy needs.
- ❑ Keep your intake of sweets and fatty foods to a minimum. These foods are low in nutrient density.
- ❑ Choose whole or unrefined grain products when possible, or use fortified or enriched cereal products.
- ❑ Use a variety of fruits and vegetables, including foods that are good sources of vitamins A and C.
- ❑ If you use milk or dairy products, choose skim or low-fat or non-fat varieties.
- ❑ Eggs are considered alright for most vegetarian diets, but one must use it with moderation. Because eggs have a high cholesterol content (213 mg per yolk), monitor your use of eggs as you try to limit your cholesterol intake to no more than 300 mg per day.

Healthful Soya

For thousands of years, populations throughout much of the world consumed soyabeans without realizing that this bean has some miraculous health properties. Today, soya has become the centre of a lot of attention. Researchers are studying the compounds found in soya that may not only help reduce the risk of some diseases, such as heart disease, osteoporosis and cancer, but also help alleviate the symptoms of menopause. Listed below are some of the more common soya foods on the market today.

Green vegetable soybeans (edamamé): These large soybeans are harvested when the beans are still green and taste sweet. They can be served as a snack or a main vegetable dish, after boiling in slightly salted water for 15 to 20 minutes. They are high in protein and fibre and contain no cholesterol. .

Meat alternatives (meat analogs): Meat alternatives (also called meat analogs) are non-meat foods made from soya protein and other ingredients mixed together to simulate various kinds of meat. Usually, they can be used the same way as the foods they replace. .

Soya cheese: Soya cheese is made from soymilk. It can substitute for sour cream or cream cheese and can be found in variety of flavours in natural-food stores.

Soya flour: Soya flour is made from roasted soyabeans that are ground into a fine powder. To turn normal wheat flour into protein packed one; mix in soya-flour, which can easily be made out of soya-bean. Soya flour is gluten-free, so yeast-raised breads made with soya flour are more dense in texture. Replace ¼ to 1/3 of the flour called for in a recipe (for chapatis, cakes, cookies, pancakes and quick breads) with soya flour.

Soya granules: Soya granules are similar to soya flour, except that the soybeans have been toasted and cracked into coarse pieces, rather than the fine powder of soya flour. Soya grits can be used as a substitute for flour in some recipes. High in protein, soya grits can be cooked together with other grains.

Soya protein isolates (isolated soya protein): When protein is removed from defatted flakes, the result is soya protein isolates. Soya protein isolates contain the most amount of protein of all soya products.

Textured soya flour (TSF): TSF is made by running defatted soya flour through an extrusion cooker, which allows for many different forms and sizes. When hydrated, it has a chewy texture. It is widely used as a meat extender. Textured soya flour contains about 70 percent protein and retains most of the bean's dietary fibre. Often referred to simply as textured soya protein (TSP), textured soya flour is sold dried in granular and chunk style.

Soya sauce: Soya sauce is a dark brown liquid made from soybeans that have undergone a fermenting process. Soya sauces have a salty taste, but are lower in sodium than traditional table salt. Soya sauce is extensively used in Chinese cuisine.

Soya yoghurt: Soya yoghurt is made from soymilk. Its creamy texture makes it an easy substitute for sour cream or cream cheese. Soya yoghurt can be found in variety of flavours in natural-food stores.

Soybeans whole: As soybeans mature in the pod, they ripen into a hard, dry bean. Most soybeans are yellow, but there are brown and black varieties. Whole soybeans (an excellent source of protein and dietary fibre) can be cooked and used in sauces, stews and soups. Whole soybeans that have been soaked can be roasted for snacks.

Soya milk, soya beverages: Soybeans, soaked, ground fine and strained, produce a fluid called soybean milk, which is a good substitute for cow's milk. Plain, unfortified soya milk is an excellent source of high-quality protein and B-vitamins.

Soya nuts: Roasted soya nuts are whole soybeans that have been soaked in water and then baked until browned. Soya nuts can be found in a variety of flavours, including chocolate. High in protein and isoflavones, soya nuts are similar in texture and flavour to peanuts.

Soya oil and products: Soya oil is the natural oil extracted from whole soybeans. Oil sold in the grocery store under the generic name "vegetable oil" is usually 100 percent soya oil or a blend of soya oil and other oils. Read the label to make certain you're buying soybean oil. Soya oil is cholesterol-free and high in polyunsaturated fat. Soya oil also is used to make margarine and shortening.

Tofu and tofu products: Tofu, also known as soybean curd, is a soft cheese-like food made by curdling fresh, hot soya milk with a coagulant. Tofu is a bland product that easily absorbs the flavours of other ingredients with which it is cooked. Tofu is rich in high-quality protein and B-vitamins and is low in sodium. Firm tofu (easy to stir fry or grill) is dense and solid and can be cubed and served in soups. Firm tofu is higher in protein, fat and calcium than other forms of tofu. Soft tofu is good for recipes that call for blended tofu. Silken tofu is a creamy product and can be used as a replacement for sour cream in many dip recipes.

Chapter **18**

DISEASE FIGHTING FOODS

The air we breathe, the water we drink and the food that we eat have a major impact on our health. A cumulative impact of toxins on our systems leads to degenerative diseases like cancer, heart diseases, diabetes, etc. Although it is one of the many factors, diet may affect your chances of getting cancer or coronary heart disease. About 50% of all cancers have been linked to diet and lifestyle factors.

The diet typical of industrialised nations has virtually eliminated diseases caused by nutritional deficiencies but the high saturated fat content of that diet is known to have detrimental effects on health. While eating a varied, balanced diet does not guarantee that you will never develop cancer or heart disease, it may well cut your risk. Certain categories of food cruciferous vegetables and food rich in beta-carotene have an especially strong protective effect. Onion and garlic have more than 30 different compounds that have anti-cancer properties. Research continues on the possible benefits of other nutrients and foods in preventing disease.

Soya beans: contain phytosterols and saponins, which stimulate immunity, slow down the growth of cancerous cells. The phytostrogens contained in soybeans may help thwart the development of hormone related cancers. Soya bean compounds also help neutralise nitrosamines, which are implicated in liver cancer.

Garlic: can help reduce blood cholesterol and triglycerides levels and maybe anti-carcinogenic. The compounds in garlic help to neutralise dangerous nitrosamines and aflatoxins which are cancer causing.

Onions: contain substances that prevent blood clots and raise HDL – cholesterol levels.

Selenium: a trace mineral may reduce cancer incidence, possibly by acting as an anti-oxidant. Seafood is a good source of selenium. Until recently, this mineral was thought to be essential for animals but harmful to humans, it is only recently that its powerful immune boosting activity has been discovered. It is a strong defence against free radicals and works best along with beta-carotene and vitamin E. Selenium helps prevent breast cancer and prostate cancer. It helps prevent strokes and hardening of arteries. Selenium is found in small quantities in whole grains, sunflower seeds, garlic, Brazil nuts, etc.

Shiitake mushrooms: these are brown or tan in colour, available, both, in fresh and dried form. They are extensively used in Chinese cooking. They contain 'Lentinan', which helps to build up immunity and reduces the side effects of chemotherapy. They also contain interferon which helps fight cancer. These mushrooms are blood thinners, they help reduce cholesterol and improve blood circulation. They are rich in immune building minerals, selenium and germanium, both of which are beneficial to prevent and fight cancer.

Green Juices: the juices extracted from wheat grass, barley grass, mint, coriander, spinach, etc., are very rich in chlorophyll, which helps to purify and cleanse the blood of toxins. Chlorophyll has powerful anti-oxidants, which help to thwart the progress of cancer. Green juices also help to balance the pH of the blood. Ideal pH range of the blood is 7.2 to 7.4. Consuming foods like maida, sugar, fried food and non-vegetarian food makes the blood more acidic and prone to diseases. Green juices keep the blood slightly alkaline, which is important for the treatment and prevention of cancer.

Sprouts: sprouted pulses like moong, moth, chana, alfa-alfa are dense in nutrients and help in keeping the blood alkaline. Brown rice and millets are alkaline cereals and beneficial in the prevention of cancer.

Vitamin E: may cut cancer and heart attack risk by acting as an anti-oxidant. Wheat germ and whole grains are good food sources.

Green vegetables and fruits: people who eat at least 6-8 servings of fruits and vegetables are less likely to get cancer. If you are genetically prone to cancer, your diet should consist of 80% alkaline forming foods such as apples, bananas, dates, figs, berries, sweet lime, watermelon, mangoes, papaya, peaches, cherries, whole grains, nuts and seeds. Freshly squeezed vegetable juices as well as fruit juices proved valuable enzymes that aid digestion. Eating these foods provides the body with the much-needed fibre, which facilitates the transit of foods through our system. The toxins therefore, do not come in contact with our GI tract for very long. This significantly reduces the risk of colorectal cancer.

Cruciferous vegetables are known to be more potent in their anti-cancer activities. This is because these are rich in 'indoles', which help in removing cancer-causing substances from the body. Vegetables like mustard, cabbage, cauliflower and broccoli fall under this category.

Omegas 3 fatty acids: from fish have an anti-inflammatory effect and may help control blood pressure and cholesterol levels.

Phytochemicals: found in fruits and vegetables may protect against cancer and heart disease.

Chapter **19**

CANCER REDUCING FOODS

It is estimated, that one third of all cancer deaths are related to diet. The following recommendations based on the national cancer institute of America may help to reduce the risk.

- Avoid obesity. It is associated with an increased risk for the cancer of the uterus, ovary, gall bladder, kidney, colon and breast.
- Cut total fat consumption. Excess fat intake may raise the risk of breast, colon and prostrate cancer.
- Eat more high fibre foods. Populations where diets are high in fibre generally have a low incidence of cancer, particularly colon cancer. Insoluble fibre is considered especially anti carcinogenic because it adds bulk to the stool and helps speed its passage through the bowel, thereby reducing the colon's exposure to potentially harmful substances in the stool. Whole grains, dried beans, and many vegetables are good source of fibre.
- Eat a variety of vegetables and fruits, especially cruciferous vegetables and foods rich in beta-carotene and vitamin C. Cruciferous vegetables named for the characteristic cross made by the four petals of their flowers, these cabbage family vegetables include broccoli, Brussels sprout, cauliflower, collard greens, kale, mustard greens as well as cabbage. They contain compounds called 'indoles' isothiocyanites, and flavones that seem to offer protection against lungs, gastro-intestinal, and other cancers.
- Beta-carotenes are a form of vitamin A. It acts as an anti oxidant, offering protection against lung cancer and reducing heart disease and stroke risk. Unlike vitamin A, beta-carotene isn't toxic in high doses. Good sources are oranges, yellow and dark green vegetables and fruits

including apricots, broccoli, cantaloupe, carrots, kale, spinach, sweet potatoes, winter squash.

- Vitamin C, in addition to acting as an anti oxidant, this vitamin may help to prevent the development of cancer, especially cancer of the oesophagus and stomach, by blocking the formation of cancer causing nitrosamine in the digestive tract. Rich sources of vitamin C are citrus fruits, strawberries, broccoli, Brussels sprouts, guavas, black currants and bell pepper.
- Limit your intake of salt, salt cured, nitrate cured and smoked foods. Nitrites and nitrates in cured foods can be converted into carcinogenic nitrosamines during cooking or in the body. The incidents of stomach and oesophageal cancers are high in countries where cured foods are eaten regularly.
- Moderate your alcohol consumption. Heavy drinking increases smokers' cancer risk, among both smokers and non smokers, heavy drinking is associated with a higher risk of cancer of the mouth, throat, oesophagus, liver and possibly breast.

Chapter 20

FOOD ADDITIVES

What Are Food Additives?

Food additives are substances that make foods last longer, taste better, look more appetising, and have a smoother consistency; some even enhance the nutritional value of food. The most common are salt, sugar and corn sweeteners.

Have you ever wondered why some peanut butters don't separate? Or why most breakfast cereals have so many vitamins and minerals? It's all due to food additives. A food additive is any substance that is used for a specific purpose in the production, processing, treatment, packaging, transportation or storage of food.

Useful Functions

For food preparation: Some additives help bread rise, keep chocolate suspended in chocolate milk, and keep seasoning blends from clumping. For example, emulsifiers give products a consistent texture and prevent them from separating.

For nutritional value: Vitamins and minerals are added to many common foods, such as milk, flour, cereal and margarine, to make them more nutritious and prevent possible health problems. Some foods are enriched with nutrients that are lost in processing. Other foods are fortified; meaning nutrients not present before processing are added. For example, vitamin A and D in milk, folic acid in some grain products, and calcium in orange juice.

For freshness and safety: Preservatives slow product spoilage caused by mould, air, bacteria, fungi or yeast. Bacterial contamination can cause food borne illness, such as botulism and salmonella poisoning. Preservatives such as antioxidants help baked goods preserve their flavour by preventing the fats and oils from becoming rancid. They also keep fresh fruits from turning brown when exposed to the air.

Many food additives contain anti-microbial agents, which inhibit the growth of micro-organisms. Flavouring and flavour enhancers may be natural substances such as salt, sugar, and spices or synthetics such as ethyl vanillin (a vanilla substitute).

For cosmetic value: Food colourings give foods a more appealing and consistent appearance. Stabilises, thickeners, and emulsifiers ensure smooth consistency and keep ingredients from spreading.

Some of them control the acidity and alkalinity, and provide leavening. Specific additives assist in modification of the acidity or alkalinity of foods to obtain a desired taste, colour, or flavour. Leavening agents that release acids when they are heated react with baking soda to help biscuits, cakes and other baked goods rise.

Are Additives Dangerous?

Most aren't. One of the most common food additives used by us is Aji-no-moto or Mono sodium glutamate. It is used to enhance food flavour, mainly in Chinese cuisine. People sensitive to MSG may have mild and transitory reactions when they eat foods that contain large amounts of MSG (such as would be found in heavily flavour-enhanced foods). Because MSG is commonly used in Chinese cuisine, these reactions were initially referred to as "Chinese restaurant syndrome."

Sulfites are used primarily as antioxidants to prevent or reduce discoloration of light-coloured fruits and vegetables, such as dried apples and potatoes, and to inhibit the growth of micro-organisms in fermented foods, such as wine. Though most people don't have a problem with sulfites, they are a hazard of unpredictable severity to people, particularly asthmatics, who are sensitive to these substances

Concern about the safety of additives has led some food processors to find safer substitutes for questionable additives. The list of controversial additives include artificial sweeteners

Precautions

Limit your intake of additives. Choose freshly or minimally processed foods over additive laden products. Eat a variety of foods to avoid ingesting too much of any single additive. Read food labels carefully; restrict your intake of foods containing artificial colours. And to keep matters in perspective, remember that too much fat or salt in your diet can be far more damaging to your health than any of the synthetic additives, currently approved for use, in our foods. The use of food additives should especially be controlled where children are concerned.

ROAD TO HEALTH CARE

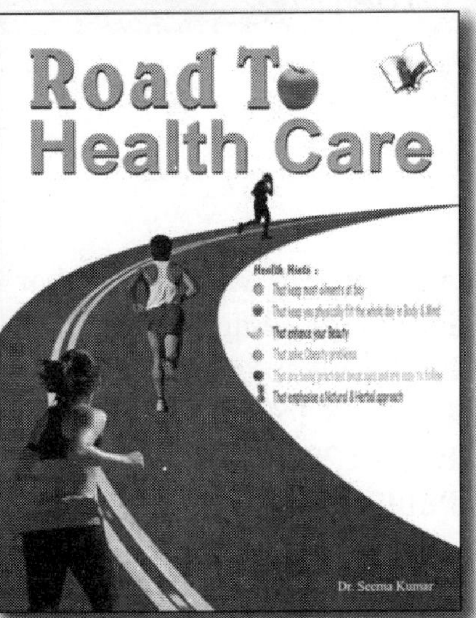

Author : Dr. Seema Kumar
Language : English
Format: Paperback
Price : ₹ 175
Pages : 176
Publisher: V&S Publishers

With ever-rising ground, water and atmospheric pollution, every other day one hears the name of a new disease. Ever since man began drifting away from Nature, he is falling into the trap of a materialistic lifestyle that has desensitised him. Today, we breathe air thick with exhaust fumes, eat processed junk food that has no nutritive value, drink toxic carbonated beverages and lead sedentary lives. All of this ensures that we are plagued with different kinds of problems at regular intervals.

This book shows you how to go back to Mother Nature to beat even the most troublesome and chronic ailments. With natural preventive measures that emphasise diet, exercise and herbal remedies, there are no fears of obnoxious side effects.

Whatever be your problem – diabetes, blood pressure, asthma, acne, menopause, obesity, stomach ailments, premature ageing or general complaints – this book shows you a safe, natural and enjoyable means to overcome it. Most of the ingredients mentioned in the book are the kind available in home gardens or off the kitchen shelf.

The book also includes hints for different stages in life. A separate section deals with varied problems in a woman's life through adolescence, pregnancy, lactation, menopause and general ailments.

Once you have read this book from cover to cover, you need not rush to the doctor every now and then, but will be able to take care of your own and your family's health yourself.

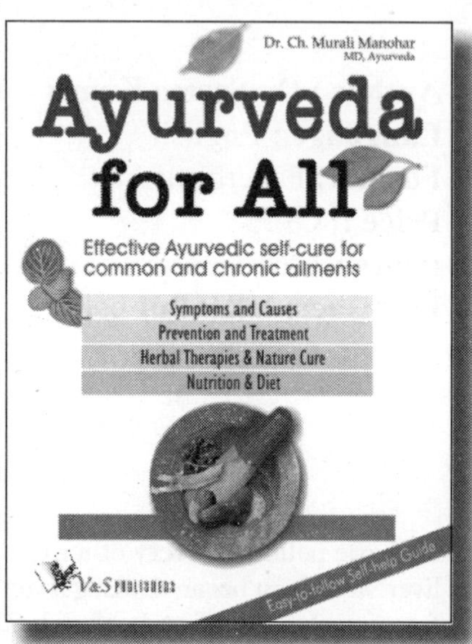

Author : Dr. Murali Manohar
Language : English
Format: Paperback
Price : ₹ 150
Pages : 220
Publisher: V&S Publishers

Recent years have seen a tremendous progress in the knowledge and practice of traditional Ayurvedic medicine, not only in India, but the world over.

Once treated with disdain, the exciting discoveries being pioneered by leading research scientists are proving that Ayurveda with its emphasis on health as well as disease is probably the world s most holistic health system.

As allopathic drugs extract a heavy toll in costs and side-effects, more and more people worldwide are turning to complementary medical systems like Ayurveda, Homeopathy, Reiki, Acupr- essure and many others.

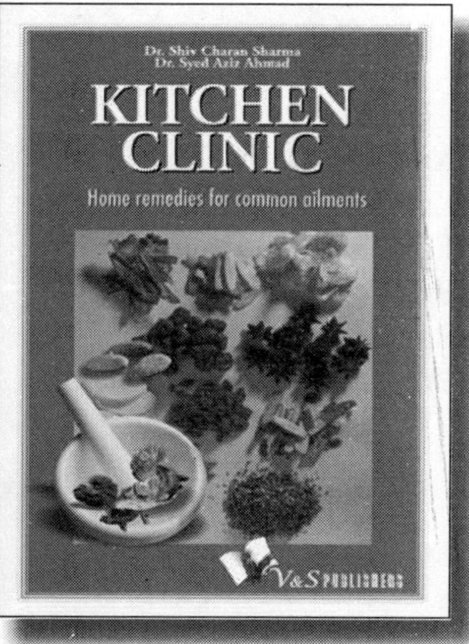

Author : Dr. Shiv Charan Sharma
Language : English
Format: Paperback
Price : ₹ 96
Pages : 150
Publisher: V&S Publishers

Home remedies and treatment of diseases by domestic plants have been prevalent since the time immemorial in India. The knowledge about the miraculous curing properties of plants is limited to certain people and is passed from one generation to another.

In the present book, the authors describe medicinal uses of 59 plants, which are used in daily life in the kitchen of Indian homes. Botanical names, vernacular names, identification, distribution and medicinal uses of each plant have been given. The book will serve as a guide of home remedies as practised by our grandmothers, in the middle of night or at odd hours when drug stores are closed. This book gives some alternate ways of controlling earaches, insomnia, minor burns, coughs, eczema, sore throats etc.

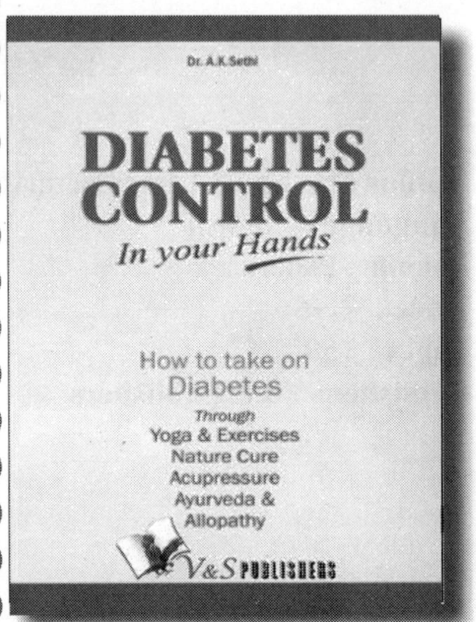

Author : Dr. A.K. Sethi
Language : English
Format: Paperback
Price : ₹ 96
Pages : 120
Publisher: V&S Publishers

Take on Diabetes through Diet-control, Yoga & Exercise, Nature Cure, Acupressure, Ayurveda and Allopathy.

Since diabetes cannot be cured, the only way to deal with it is to learn how to control it. With this clear objective in view, the book offers a complete guide on the ways and means to go about it.

Where the book scores over others is that it does not just confine itself to Allopathic treatment but offers a complete controlling mechanism covering Ayurveda, Yoga, Nature Cure, Acupressure, Feng Shui through conventional and non-conventional ways.

This book is a must not only for those affected by diabetes, but everyone above forty who could run the risk of getting it.

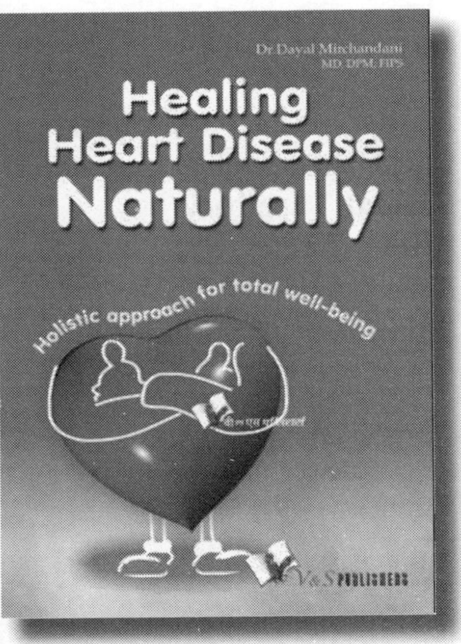

Author : Dr. Dayal Mirchandani
Language : English
Format: Paperback
Price : ₹ 96
Pages : 200
Publisher: V&S Publishers

Recent advances in the behavioural sciences have ensured that a variety of physical disorders can be healed using psychological techniques.

In fact, worldwide, mind-body healing is being increasingly used to treat chronic illnesses such as asthma, ulcerative colitis, rheumatoid arthritis and coronary artery disease with excellent results.

This book reveals the personality trait that puts you at highest risk and how to change it, how to use self-hypnosis and imagery in healing your heart, how to stop smoking permanently with little or no discomfort, how to find meaning and joy in life, besides other practical techniques to reverse heart disease.

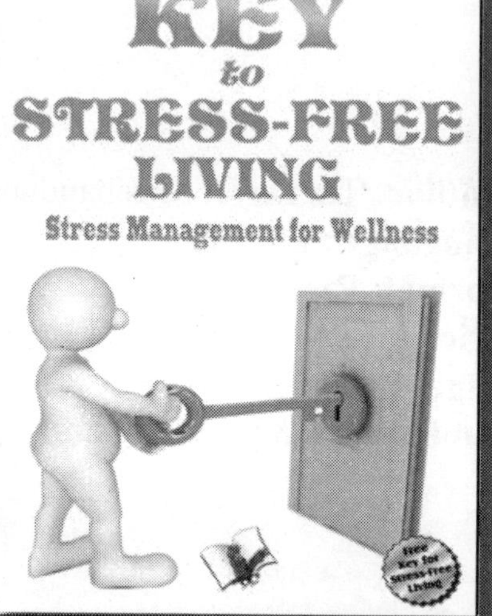

Free Keychain

Author : Dr. Jyotsna Codaty
Language : English
Format: Paperback
Price : ₹ 150
Pages : 136
Publisher: V&S Publishers

There are three primary aspects of life that contribute to promoting unhealthy stress which ultimately kills – inability to make decisions, feeling lack of control in life, and not having a plan or process in place to get to where you need to go. Spread over 18 chapters, this book has put together all the necessary materials to take control of your life, make wise decisions, and be proactive in taking care of things that typically stress you out. This book contains principles and ideas that will go a long way in reducing the stress that people have in this 21st century.

The fact that you are reading the blurb of a book on stress management, maybe out of sheer curiosity, signifies that you are trying to decipher if life could be made more meaningful and positive, no matter how contented or stressful life you are leading at the moment. This book is full of tips worth reading, especially given the author's credentials.

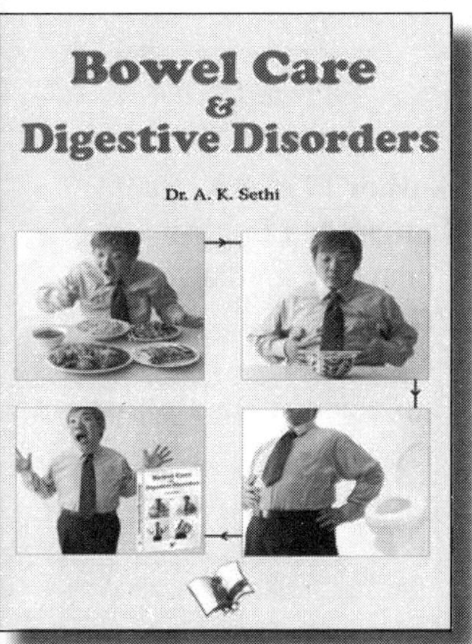

Author : Dr. A.K. Sethi
Language : English
Format: Paperback
Price : ₹ 135
Pages : 132
Publisher: V&S Publishers

Most people are shy about discussing Bowel care & Digestive Disorders, but few realize how important it is. The truth is that it needs utmost care and attention. The bowel has very few nervous leads- otherwise you would feel the digestion and bowel movement all day long. So, if you feel you have a digestive problem of sorts, you better attend to it immediately.

Most toxins enter our body through the digestive tract, along with our food and drinks. If we don't eat healthy, we tend to accumulate toxic wastes resulting in increased bowel transit time, and the wastes, instead of getting eliminated, stay put inside our body. These wastes, putrefy further and become a breeding ground for harmful bacteria and other parasites which in turn leads to more serious diseases and problems developing in the body.

This book is an authoritative reference source on bowel care and digestive disorders of various types. Written in a very convincing and captivating manner providing some anatomy lessons about the digestive tract, causes and symptoms of bowel disorders (constipation, diarrhea, etc.), the book lists proper diagnosis and treatment. It has been designed as an ideal self-help guide through yoga, meditation, ayurvedic treatment and alternative treatment methods like magneto therapy, acupressure, colour therapy, vastu, aromatherapy and music therapy to manage bowel disorders.

HOW TO HAVE SOUND SLEEP

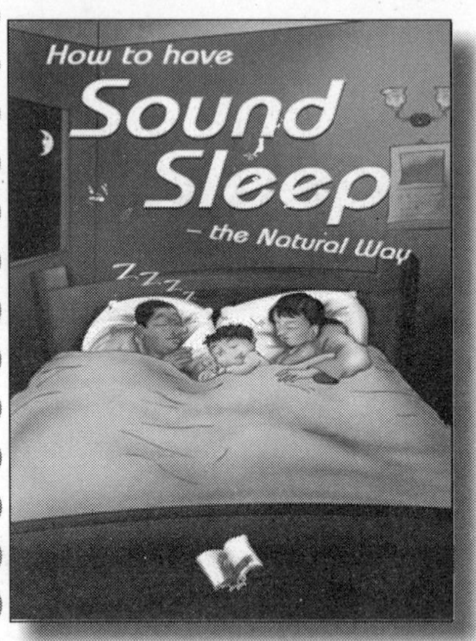

Author : Dr. A.K. Sethi
Language : English
Format: Paperback
Price : ₹ 135
Pages : 136
Publisher: V&S Publishers

Sleep Deprivation Can Make You Obese, Forgetful, Aged and Diseased for the Rest of Your Life!

Don't blame lifestyle for your disturbed sleep. Did you know that sleeping more or fewer than seven hours a day greatly impairs the production of thyroid and stress hormones. This impairment, in turn, not only affects the memory, immune system and metabolism etc., but also increases the risk of high blood sugar levels, hypertension (high blood pressure), weight gain, accelerated ageing, depression and increased risk of heart attack.

Researchers have also determined that sleeping adequately after a few days of disturbed sleep can very nearly erase any lingering sense of mental haziness and fatigue. In order to help you get a sound sleep and also to protect you from the need to take recourse to making up any lost sleep or disorder, the book details the importance, benefits, physiology and body reinvigoration of having sound sleep, untoward effects of sleep disorders and natural & non-conventional methods of managing it. Also explained in various chapters are advantages of proper exercise, yoga, naturopathy, acupressure, colour & music therapy, lifestyle changes etc., that enable waking up in the morning feeling fresh, fit and trim. A separate chapter is devoted to the Dos and Don'ts to highlight factors that contribute towards bringing sound sleep.

An indispensible book guaranteeing Sound Sleep to all readers every night!

All books available at www.vspublishers.com

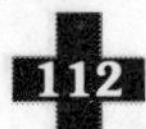